Reflexology

Chris Stormer

TEACH YOURSELF BOOKS

For UK orders: please contact Bookpoint Ltd, 39 Milton Park, Abingdon, Oxon OX14 4TD. Telephone: (44) 01235 400414, Fax: (44) 01235 400454. Lines are open from 9.00 – 6.00, Monday to Saturday, with a 24 hour message answering service. Email address: orders@bookpoint.co.uk

For U.S.A. & Canada orders: please contact NTC/Contemporary Publishing, 4255 West Touhy Avenue, Lincolnwood, Illinois 60646 – 1975, U.S.A.. Telephone: (847) 679 5500, Fax: (847) 679 2494.

Long-renowned as the authoritative source for self-guided learning – with more than 30 million copies sold worldwide – the *Teach Yourself* series includes over 200 titles in the fields of languages, crafts, hobbies, business and education.

British Library Cataloguing in Publication Data
A catalogue record for this title is available from The British Library

Library of Congress Catalog Card Number:

First published in UK 1996 by Hodder Headline Plc, 338 Euston Road, London NW1 3BH

First published in US 1996 by NTC/Contemporary Publishing, 4255 West Touhy Avenue, Lincolnwood (Chicago), Illinois 60646 – 1975 U.S.A.

The 'Teach Yourself' name and logo are registered trade marks of Hodder & Stoughton Ltd.

Copyright © 1996 Chris Stormer

Typeset by Transet Limited, Coventry, England.
Printed in Great Britain for Hodder & Stoughton Educational, a division of Hodder Headline Plc, 338 Euston Road, London NW1 3BH by Cox & Wyman Ltd, Reading, Berkshire.

Impression number	15	14	13	12	11	10	9	8	7	6
Year		2005	2004	2003	2002	2001	2000	1999		

CONTENTS

ACKNOWLEDGEMENTS

My sincere thanks to the publishers, Hodder Headline, for inviting me to write this book. I have thoroughly enjoyed the opportunity of sharing knowledge of reflexology in a slightly different manner from my previous books.

As always, none of this would have been possible without the incredible love and support of my family, particularly my wonderful man, John Fryer, and my two outstanding sons, Andrew and David. The depth of my affection and appreciation can never be adequately expressed in words.

Thanks to the tremendous loyalty and dedication of Liz Harris, my secretary, and Veronica Polo Polo, my maid, the Reflexology Academy of South Africa (RASA) is growing from strength to strength and both the Academy and home are well cared for.

My gratitude to **all** tutors, therapists and students of RASA for enriching my life, as well as generously sharing individual expertise and universal knowledge, much of which has been passed on in this book to assist others to help themselves.

To the readers, if it were not for the enlightened desire for personal development, books like this would not be possible.

May abundant happiness and ultimate fulfilment be yours.

Running Water – Thank You!

INTRODUCTION

Teach Yourself Reflexology is an easy-to-follow guide to a natural, effective and safe form of healing.

The brief background of its origins, how it works and what to expect during and after the massage provides insight into this fascinating, ancient therapy.

Simple step-by-step instructions of the soothing yet exhilarating technique will guide you reassuringly through the massage and manipulation of both feet, section by section:

- the *toes* to ease the *mind*
- the *toe necks* to open the avenues of two-way *expression*
- the *balls of the feet* to pacify the *emotions*
- the *insteps* for *inner harmony*
- the *heels* for *personal growth and development*
- the *corresponding parts* for *overall equilibrium*.

The illustrations accompanying the instructions are my own sketches. I wanted to include them in the hope that their natural simplicity will facilitate understanding of the beautiful gift of reflexology that is everyone's birthright.

From the basis provided, you can, with experience and comprehension, expand and develop your own unique approach.

Reflexology is exceptionally accommodating and it **does not matter** if, initially, attempts are slow, cumbersome, inaccurate or confused. The body naturally compensates for any perceived inadequacy.

It is impossible to cause harm, even in inexperienced hands.

Furthermore, an understanding of how inner emotions and thoughts are constantly displayed through the ever-changing characteristics of the feet will dispel any fear, especially of massaging the feet of temporarily imbalanced, unwell souls.

More common ailments that respond particularly well to the reflexology massage are also mentioned. Revelations are included of how adjustment of thoughts, feelings and actions can transform the state of mind, body and soul from being fraught, uptight and uneasy into feeling totally relaxed, flexible and healthy.

Reflexology is truly remarkable in the way in which it helps us and others to a more fulfilling, rewarding and better way of life. It is a marvel that an amazing new reality can be moulded through the sensitive massage and manipulation of a pair of feet.

❛ We have the greatest power of all – the ability to heal ourselves. ❜

1

AN EXPLANATION OF REFLEXOLOGY

A general overview

Reflexology is the firm but gentle massage and manipulation of reflexes in both feet to:

- relax the body
- ease the mind and
- reassure the soul.

Stimulation of latent healing abilities within the body creates a healthy, harmonious state, ideal for efficient physical, emotional and intellectual functioning of the whole.

This natural form of healing has stood the test of time as an ancient, non-invasive, simple and safe therapy. It is still responsible for remarkable reactions experienced worldwide today.

Reflexology massage arouses and fine-tunes *reflexes* throughout the body, since all bodily parts, organs and glands are accurately and clearly *reflected* onto the feet. Touching a specific *reflex* on the feet can, therefore, evoke a favourable, involuntary *reflex* response in the corresponding *reflected* part of the body. The feet also truthfully *reflect* the state of the mind, body and soul through the condition of the feet.

The sudden surge of vibrant energy from reflexology massage rejuvenates the physical body by flushing away emotional impediments and establishing a state of inner peace. In this way, a natural state of health can either be regained or retained.

For the healthy person, reflexology offers:

- a pleasant form of deep relaxation
- relief from fear, anxiety and frustration
- rejuvenation that re-energises mind, body and soul
- increased vitality and confidence
- improved quality of sleep
- trust in personal attributes and those of others
- prolonged acute concentration
- a feeling of incredible well-being
- restored balance
- a sense of wholeness
- a more fulfilling and rewarding experience of life and health
- the courage to cope beneficially with perceived adversity
- the confidence to express openly the true self with unconditional love and honesty
- an opportunity for personal transformation, growth and individual development.

For the less healthy, reflexology:

- relieves dis-ease at root level
- counteracts fatigue
- soothes nervousness, anxiety and fear
- eases aches, pains and discomfort
- alleviates distress
- reduces tension by relaxing the musculature
- improves circulation
- cleanses the whole of threatening substances and impurities
- stimulates sluggish, inactive areas
- calms hyperactive, over-productive parts.

The advantages of learning reflexology are that:

- anyone and everyone from toddlers onwards can administer it, provided there is an interest
- it can be applied at any time, or in any situation, since the only essential requirements are the hands of the masseur and the feet of the recipient
- academic achievements not essential
- medical knowledge is useful but **not** necessary
- only the feet are exposed, reducing embarrassment, self-consciousness and possible vulnerability

- painful bodily parts are left undisturbed, yet relief can still be obtained by applying reflexology on the related reflex in the feet
- with less skin surface on the feet than on the body, a more thorough and precise massage is possible.

Acquiring knowledge of reflexology is fascinating, enjoyable and rewarding. With no right or wrong ways to apply reflexology, understanding of applied principles is facilitated.

Although a reflexology massage takes an hour, its effects last much longer, with favourable reactions, even from sceptics. This is because reflexology is one of the most encompassing and wholistic disciplines of healing known to mankind.

6 Health and healing are only two feet away! 9

History and background

Reflexology is an ancient and gentle form of healing that has been passed from generation to generation for centuries. When humans first placed their feet on the earth's surface, they were naturally stimulated by walking and running over the uneven ground, but the introduction of sandals and shoes has diminished their inborn sensitivity.

Throughout history feet have represented mobility, security and grounding. According to Greek legend, the feet symbolised the soul, with any lameness being perceived as weakness of spirit, whilst in ancient Egypt, 'soles' of feet were removed, during mummification, to liberate the 'soul' from physical bondage and commitment to the earth plane.

Witches, on being declared guilty, were immediately raised from the ground, to sever all contact with Mother Earth, the source from which, it was believed, mystical powers were absorbed through the feet.

Until AD 200, many flocked to the Delphi health resort in Greece to relax in the sacred waters of the hydrotherapy pools. Before retiring to a sleep temple, reflexology and body massage were administered to evoke memories and foresight through dreams. Interpretation of these visions provided guidance and direction.

According to Japanese mythology, a wise old soul, called Outo, when questioned about his incredible healing powers, replied:

> 'See to the feet, my friend, and you have seen to the body.'
> 'I do not understand,' protested the bewildered investigator.
> Otou responded: 'Your understanding will never be enough. See to the feet, that is all that is required.'

Otou was aware that feet reveal all, on every level.

Reflexology is synonymous with the symbolic ritual of welcome and purification through the anointment, washing and massage of feet, of which there are over 33 references in the Bible. Reflexology, as an act of acceptance, encourages mind, body and soul to cleanse and purify themselves through the elimination of toxic substances.

Kissing and worshipping the feet of divine or eminent people as a sign of respect has been evident in most cultures worldwide. It is still practised in certain rural parts of India, where youngsters embrace their parents' feet as a sign of love and appreciation.

Today many travel to India seeking the opportunity to glimpse or touch the feet of devout, spiritual men, such as Sai Baba, to attain inner peace and personal enlightenment. Gathering dust from their footsteps has brought further illumination and serenity to numerous believers.

Over the years, countless people have eventually found relief from extreme discomfort by turning to reflexology when other methods have failed. Following an assassination attempt, the twentieth President of the United States of America, President Garfield (1831–81) continued to suffer excruciating pain despite endless sophisticated forms of treatment until, in desperation, he turned to reflexology and finally discovered exceptional ease and increased comfort.

Reflexology is a self-help therapy that provides natural healing for everyone, regardless of skin colour or religious conviction. Its simplicity and uncomplicated effectiveness in harmonising the whole reinstates reflexology as an all-encompassing healing therapy that keeps individuals in 'good working order'.

> ❻ Roots and foundations provide a firm basis for personal growth and development – if restricted, potential is inhibited – whereas liberation frees individuals to venture forth unimpeded. ❾

Complementing one another:
modern medicine and reflexology

Orthodox medicine, at around 300 years old, is relatively young compared to complementary healing methods. Reflexology dates back to the beginning of human life when reflexes in the feet were naturally stimulated by walking and running barefoot over the earth's undulating surfaces.

Invaluable insight and understanding of bodily organs and functions, through medical research, have allowed ancient healing methods to expand and be effectively adapted to meet the ever-changing, progressive needs of present society.

Interestingly, progressive development and sophistication of the mind are continually reflected through enlarging characteristics of the body and feet as individuals are willing to become greater beings and make a larger impression and impact on life.

Hippocrates, the acknowledged Father of Medicine, believed that detection of fluctuating bodily humours and ever-changing physical conditions revealed the emotion responsible for the mind's disposition. Through this study, the most appropriate remedy could be determined.

The state of the body reflects the mood and perceptions of the mind with:

- health revealing ease of mind and inner peace
- dis-ease being an outward manifestation of inner emotional conflict or turmoil.

Balance between health and dis-ease is easily and temptingly tipped by an unhealthy obsession with physical, materialistic aspects that deprive mind, body and soul of ultimate fulfilment on the earth plane. Impoverished self-esteem and self-worth are evident through perceived poverty and personal denial.

> ❝ For complete harmony and health, there must be enrichment of mind, body and soul. ❞

Modern technology is incredible. Used advantageously, it provides liberation from mundane tasks to allow more time for personal pursuits. Utilisation of unique individual skills and talents encourages personal growth and self-development. If these opportunities are overlooked or ignored, resulting discontent, uneasiness, frustration and bewilderment will invariably cause inner turmoil and emotional conflict. This is evident in widespread dis-eases throughout the world today.

Modern medicine caters for bodily and intellectual needs by offering solutions that ease physical pain and discomfort. These stepping stones, if used advantageously, can bridge the gap between the symptoms of physical dis-ease and emotional distress. However, for complete relief from discomfort and illness a complete shift of thought and change of attitude are essential since lives are a product of perceptions. For example, increased sensitivity causes irritability, highlighted through skin rashes; increased mucus production and hypersensitivity will continue until replaced by a more tolerant outlook on life. Placebos, tablets without drug content, are used effectively as antidotes because of the conviction with which they are administered and received. The mind's belief becomes the body's reality.

Reflexology encourages natural healing of mind, body and soul at a subconscious level, without having to stir past traumatic memories. Further emotional havoc and distress can, therefore, be avoided. It is not possible to re-align broken bones through reflexology but, through relaxation induced by this natural therapy, discomfort can be eased and the healing process accelerated.

Modern medical knowledge has provided reflexology and other forms of complementary healing with the incentive to take healing a step further. Just as bodily symptoms reflect the state of mind, so the condition of feet accurately display the emotions and feelings behind disease, consciously, subconsciously and unconsciously. Specific individual needs can then be comprehended, revealing the power of this ancient but amazing natural therapy.

Reflexology and modern medicine, used beneficially together, are a dynamic combination. With a more wholistic approach to healing, medical professionals in hospitals worldwide are recognising the need to employ reflexology therapists to ease stress-related disorders and assist in speeding up the recovery process. Results to date have been phenomenal.

Reflexology therapy and modern medicine are an ideal combination of sophisticated modern technology and ancient knowledge and wisdom.

> ‘Competition and comparisons are futile, for individuals are intentionally unique to encourage personal growth and development through the exchange and sharing of ideas and concepts.’

Other forms of complementary healing

Natural healing mediums provide an array of therapies and remedies on which the mind, body and soul can thrive.

The *Alexander technique* realigns bodily posture to balance the musculature and re-energise the whole. Reflexology can enhance the effect of this procedure by easing tension and relaxing the muscles.

Aromatherapy uses the evocative sense of aromatic smell, often combined with oils, to be massaged onto the skin and absorbed into the body for relaxation and overall harmony. Using these exquisite oils on the feet, either during or after reflexology, accelerates healing. Try this popular combination:

Bergamot to calm nerves
Neroli to boost self-confidence
Ylang-ylang to heighten the senses
Juniper to assist in detoxification.

Refer to Appendix I for the properties of other aromatherapy oils.

Bach, Findhorn and *Australian Flower Remedies* are natural extracts from the plant kingdom that create inner strength and deeper understanding to cope with persistent draining thoughts or mood swings. Taken orally between reflexology massages, soul-destroying cycles become less threatening and more manageable. A bottle of Rescue Remedy, which is a combination of five potent remedies, is essential for times of extreme distress or shock since it immediately encourages a state of inner peace.

Colour healing balances the finely tuned body, by equalising personal vibrations through the resonance of various colours. During a reflexology massage, visualisation of specific hues alters the tone of mind, body and soul to harmonise the whole.

See Appendix II for the healing properties of colours.

Crystals and other gems, universally popular as beautiful adornments, have also been recognised throughout the Ages for their potent healing properties. Rose quartz held loosely in each hand during reflexology can encourage self-acceptance and may fill the whole with renewed vibrancy. The effect may be enhanced by gently placing the stones on the solar plexus reflexes at the end of the massage.

Herbs, used extensively in cooking, have numerous remedial qualities, the secrets of which have been passed from generation to generation. Herbs, as a natural source of energy, complement reflexology in preserving health.

Homoeopathy and *naturopathy* alleviate dis-ease through natural derivatives. Healing can be accentuated by using these panacea between reflexology sessions.

Music during reflexology can be exceptionally therapeutic:

● Gregorian chants create inner calm
● Mozart's music is rich in high frequencies and fills the whole with vibrancy and enthusiasm
● Dolphin and whale music can be remarkably calming and reassuring, particularly for:
  – pregnant women
  – children
  – dis-eased souls
  – the autistic
  – the unconscious.

See Appendix III for suggested healing music.

Reiki shifts and balances bodily vibrations by directing life-forces from the hands, particularly the fingertips, of the administrator to areas of the body that lack energy and vitality. These intensified healing energies and vibrations can empower the outcome of a reflexology massage.

Shiatsu, acupressure and *acupuncture* clear vital energy pathways for the penetration of natural life-forces to all bodily cells.

❢ Artificial remedies provide unnatural, temporary reactions, unless accompanied by a change of mind. Natural remedies naturally relieve and ease mind, body and soul. ❵

2
THE ROLE OF
REFLEXOLOGY

Ease or dis-ease

A healthy person feels fantastic, wakes up energised, enjoys the challenges and opportunities, enthuses about pursuits and appreciates the gift of life. This is **living**! The quality of personal circumstances depends on whether emotions are in tune or in conflict with the natural flow of life-forces, which then determines the state of ease or dis-ease.

Health outwardly manifests peace of mind, body and soul, whereas disease displays feelings of being ill at ease from trying to live up to the expectations of others. The isolation of the body and mind from the soul's purpose causes frustration, bewilderment, doubt, unhappiness and emotional loneliness.

A perceived need to conform to limited, often outdated, belief systems robs individuals of unique talents resulting in distress, pressure and tension. This can:

- hamper progress
- interfere with performance
- cause overreaction to minor situations
- give rise to inappropriate anger or impatience
- increase or decrease the appetite
- lead to abusive use of
  - alcohol to drown sorrows
  - food to cover up the true self or provide protection from perceived maltreatment

– tobacco to create a smokescreen and conceal soulful emotions
– drugs to desensitise personal turmoil.

A dis-eased person is a potentially healthy person temporarily imbalanced and out of sync with natural life-forces. The physical symptoms of distress signal unhappiness and dissatisfaction.

It is natural to consciously or unconsciously want to be whole and healthy, but harmful extremes can immediately tip the balance. A distressing thought is capable of toppling even the most healthy person, whilst bizarre or outdated ideas and belief systems distort the mind and body to the detriment of personal growth and development.

Dis-ease can be an ideal time for individual development when the knocks of life are viewed as knocks of opportunity. The greater the knock, the greater the opportunity. Discovery of untapped resources and inner strengths unveil true aspects of oneself and personal abilities. With renewed meaning and direction, there is abundant energy and enthusiasm for the exciting adventure of unique discovery.

Body language, verbalised in everyday speech, is vividly reflected through characteristics of the feet:

● *Ill at ease* – tense, uptight soles
● *Injured* – dents reveal hurt pride, whilst various shades of blue to black indicate the intensity of bruised feelings
● *Upset* – feet lack composure
● *Invalid* – devoid of strength and energy
● *Off colour* – feet drained of vibrancy displaying an assortment of colours, predominantly white
● *Weak* – skin and feet lack strength and substance
● *Troubled* – concern and uneasiness displayed through wrinkled, lined skin on the feet
● *Disabled* – unable to move ahead due to an impediment
● *Distorted* – feet contorted from trying to fit into unsuitable or unfashionable belief systems.

The underlying circumstances of dis-ease differ considerably for each individual. However, the body has marvellous natural recuperative abilities that come to the fore in a relaxed, favourable environment induced by reflexology massage.

Healthy people feed the mind with loving thoughts, which clear the pathway to success. Each day is perceived to be an opportunity to do something worthwhile, with an enthusiasm and ingenuity that defies restrictions to the joy of mind, body and soul.

❝ Life is easy for those with no preferences. ❞

Defusing distress

Distress can be deadly when long-term mental anguish causes internal emotional turmoil and havoc. Inadequate functioning or breakdown of bodily cells may result in any of the following possible outcomes:

- Ulcers which eat away at supporting tissue through frustration at the lack of encouragement
- Hypertension from accumulated pressure of unresolved emotional conflicts
- Heart dis-ease due to:
  – insufficient unconditional love for oneself and others
  – hardening the heart against the bounty of life in preference for material possessions
  – fear and anxiety that squeeze the tissue and cause pain
  – personal abuse and attack
- Strokes from relentlessly trying to control everything and everyone
- Kidney failure from overwhelming disappointment.

Massaging reflex points in the feet stimulates the body's natural healing resources to overcome any minor or major symptom of distress, no matter how long standing. Vibrant life-forces are directed along natural pathways to untangle energy knots and emotional congestion.

A renewed surge of vital energy invigorates the whole by flushing out harmful lifestyle patterns and removing all impediments and any lethargy. Without pressure, the relaxed mind, body and soul can function appropriately, effectively and expansively.

The chain reaction of reflexology in combating distress and dis-ease worldwide is impressive. Continual use of this ancient form of healing to regain and retain health could result in a phenomenal decrease of heart attacks, strokes, mental disorders, suicides, accidents and hospital expenses.

Relaxation liberates mind, body and soul from the pressurising issues of perceived harsh realities of life. By gaining access to all levels, physical, mental, emotional and spiritual, reflexology can lift the whole from self-imposed limitations.

❛ Dis-ease is solely and purely corrective. ❜

Feet!

Feet provide a solid foundation for flexible mobility, personal growth and individual development. Like roots, they afford security and stability, but have the added advantage of being able to adapt to unexpected, new experiences encountered throughout life's journey.

Fear, uncertainty and anxiety tend to 'root feet to the ground' or 'allow the grass to grow under the feet'. Rigid, unhappy, insecure soles continually 'test the way', being 'unsure of their footing', making life appear arduous and heavy going.

Secure, contented people on the other hand enjoy 'standing on their own two feet', 'with a foot in the door' and 'step ahead with confidence' in a relaxed and easy manner. With 'a spring in the feet' and natural flexibility, soles are effective shock absorbers, with ankles adjusting readily to life's ups and downs.

The frequent use of the words 'foot' or 'feet' in describing a person's standing or situation in life is symbolic, reiterating the importance of their role. Here are a few commonly used sayings:

To land on one's feet –	To secure a fortunate position.
To find one's feet –	To settle down.
To put the best foot forward –	To make a good impression.
To put one's foot down –	To take a firm stand.
To put one's foot in it –	To make a *faux pas*.
To trample underfoot –	To oppress or treat with contempt.
To be on good footing –	To be on friendly terms.

Feet provide a basic understanding of individual requirements. They also display personal talents that, if realised, can fill the world with vibrancy and joy.

When feet are relaxed the rest of the body has the potential to be healthy. This is where reflexology steps in.

❝ The soles of the feet accurately reflect and provide insight into the state of the mind and needs of the soul. ❞

— **Who benefits from reflexology?** —

Anyone and everyone can benefit from reflexology's amazing ability to harmonise all bodily systems. It effectively enhances the functioning of mind, body and soul. As a relaxation technique, reflexology:

- calms the body
- releases muscular tension
- creates space for healing to occur
- naturally stimulates sluggish, hypo-active glands and organs
- soothes over-excited, hyperactive bodily parts.

With gentle, sensitive application it is impossible to cause harm with reflexology.

Be wary, however, of massaging the feet of a deep vein thrombosis sufferer who experiences excruciating pain from a blood clot in a deep vein, usually in the legs. As muscles relax their grip on the circulatory system through reflexology, the blood clot *may* dislodge and travel to the brain or heart, with the remote possibility of a stroke or heart attack. Although there has been no report of such an occurrence, it is advisable to be cautious.

Reflexology is particularly effective during:

Pregnancy
- A mother-to-be can enjoy vibrant energy and inner peace
- The relaxed womb expands more readily to accommodate the baby and creates a calm environment for the healthy growth and development of new life
- There is sufficient space for foetal movement within the uterus
- The lively circulation nourishes both mother and baby
- Vital energy can abound throughout
- There is a stronger bond of trust and unconditional love for one another.

Childhood
- Babies and children are exceptionally sensitive to parental thoughts and feelings, which are subconsciously manifested through the

health of the offspring long before the parent is aware of their own ease or dis-ease
- The well-being of youngsters improves and is maintained when parents receive reflexology since there is an increased likelihood of harmony and ease within the home
- Physical, emotional and spiritual ties between children and adults are strengthened
- Encourages personal individuality.

Adolescence
- Balances hormonal production and distribution for inner harmony
- A more trusting and honest relationship within the self and amongst others is created
- Adds confidence and impetus to step into adulthood with increased tolerance and poise.

Adult years
- Easiness of the mind is reflected in a healthier condition of the body
- Wrinkles of concern are less likely to leave their mark, with renewed faith in the process of life
- Weight taken off the mind makes the body less prone to sagging
- Reflexology encourages a more lenient, open-minded attitude
- Self-induced pressures are eased
- The damaging effect of distress, fear and anxiety is minimised.

Golden years
- Prevents mind, body and soul from withering and wasting away due to lack of enthusiasm or purpose in life, regardless of age, by injecting the whole with renewed enthusiasm
- Alerts the mind and improves concentration
- Preserves the body by keeping it in good working order through the continual replacement of worn out cells with billions of new, healthy, vibrant cells, every second of each day, in a naturally relaxed environment.

Illness
- The need for touch and reflexology increases during periods of ill health, vulnerability and defencelessness to soothe the distress and relieve symptoms of uneasiness
- Elimination of harmful substances and emotions, through natural channels within the mind and body, makes space for healthy, rejuvenated cells

- Pain and discomfort are eased by calming the mind, relaxing the body and reassuring the soul.

Within a family unit
- Bridges the gap between the generations
- Strengthens the bond between parents, children and siblings
- Encourages acceptance and understanding of personal attributes
- Creates respect and space for individual uniqueness.

   ❻ Health and healing are only possible when there is unity and harmony through peace of mind, a relaxed body and a contented soul. ❾

3

A CLOSER LOOK AT REFLEXOLOGY

How reflexology works

Uneasiness from protracted fear, anxiety and distrust causes tension that interferes with natural bodily processes. The greater the uneasiness, the greater the tension and the more damaging the interference. Distressing thoughts alarm the body which, defensively, prepares itself for an attack:

- the musculature becomes physically uptight
- tense, contracted muscles clamp down on organs and glands reducing the amount of space in which to function
- rigidity inhibits mobility
- depleted blood supplies starve bodily cells of nutritional sustenance, denying them the opportunity to grow and develop to their full capacity
- potentially dangerous toxic substances accumulate and are entrapped by the narrowed lumen of the veins and lymphatic vessels, creating unnecessary swellings and burdens.

These unnatural conditions reflect uneasiness within the mind and are displayed through symptoms of distress and dis-ease, that signal the need for beneficial action.

Pain is a desperate plea from distressed, deprived cells to the brain begging for the tension to be eased so that vital substances can get through to nourish the whole. Instead of alleviating the situation by relaxing and letting go, fear and misunderstanding cause panic and further strain, affecting neighbouring cells and spreading the dis-ease.

Prolonged tension denies affected cells space and nutrients, causing malfunctioning and eventually malformation. The latter condition is more commonly known as cancer.

Reflexology, as a relaxation technique, dissipates tension and pressure, and ultimately dis-ease. As muscles relax their tight grip:

- increased elasticity allows for greater flexibility and mobility as well as the natural expansion and contraction of bodily activity
- the uninhibited blood flow generously replenishes all bodily cells
- well-nurtured cells have the space to function and rejuvenate themselves with ease
- any potential threat from waste products or toxic substances is effectively eliminated
- a weight is lifted off the mind, body and soul
- the natural environment created is ideal for efficient functioning of the whole and for promotion of health.

Reflexology soothes from the inside out and is an impressive antidote to distress. The recipient drifts into a deeply relaxing and blissful state of alpha consciousness. During this tranquil phase that naturally occurs between wakefulness and sleep, mind, body and soul can fully recuperate.

Every second, billions of new cells are formed throughout the body so that it is kept in good working order and continually undergoes complete rejuvenation. The favourable conditions induced by reflexology allow this natural process to proceed unhindered.

A relaxed body can re-energise itself through the absorption of abundant universal energy that is obtained from two main sources:

- vibrant, positive, light sun energies are received from the surrounding atmosphere through bodily hairs that act like antennae
- solid, dark, negative earth energies are drawn in through the soles of the feet.

These energies penetrate and surround the body, mind and soul to replenish the whole with abundant vitality. Organs and glands can then vibrate with abundant energy which is reflected back onto the body's surface, particularly the feet, to radiate health. When distressed the feet may reveal:

- rigidity due to insecurity
- hardness or lack of substance from vulnerability or perceived deprivation

● weakness and exhaustion that drains the whole of vibrancy.

Heavy, unhappy thoughts, from doubt and uncertainty, weigh heavily on the mind and body, with a similar heaviness and lifelessness in the feet. Reflexology encourages the subconscious release of burdensome thoughts and emotions. Stored fears and anxieties from childhood and the past are put into perspective and no longer appear so threatening to personal well-being.

A relaxed physical body lets go on all levels, physically, mentally, emotionally and spiritually. The person consequently feels better and can think more clearly.

❝ All perceived adversities, large or small, can either destroy or be used advantageously for personal growth and development. ❞

——— Position of the reflexes ———

Reflexology has been passed from generation to generation over many centuries so it is inevitable that some reflex positions may differ slightly according to individual interpretation. The assortment of foot charts available are basically the same, with the main variations being found in the reflexes of the spine, ears, eyes, heart, breast and knee.

Since several organs, glands and vessels overlap in the body, there may be more than one reflex on a particular area of the foot. Primary reflexes access the reflected part directly, whilst secondary reflexes have an indirect approach. For example, the breast reflexes are reflected directly onto the balls of the feet, whilst secondary or indirect reflexes are situated directly opposite on top of both feet (Figure 1).

It is possible to see how perfectly all bodily parts are reflected by simply visualising a miniature version of the body's anatomy on the feet (Figure 2, pages 22–23):

● each foot represents half the body
● the front of the body is mirrored onto the soles of the feet
● the back of the body is depicted on the tops of the feet
● the right side of the body is reflected onto the right foot
● the left foot corresponds with the left side of the body.

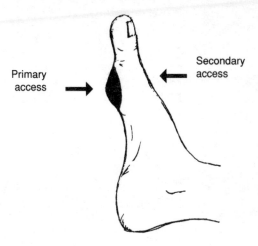

Figure 1 The primary and secondary breast reflexes

The accuracy of this is so great that:

- missing or removed bone, organ or gland, have a corresponding gap in the related part of the feet, unless scar tissue is present, in which case a matching hardness may be detected
- extra bones and organs rebound in the reflected position
- shattered reflexes of crushed bone feel splintered or gritty in the feet.

With the soles of the feet situated side by side, visualise the following bodily parts, on a substantially smaller scale:

- The cushioned pads on the toes represent the face and the many facets of the brain. Big toes placed together resemble the shape of the head and face
- Toe necks mirror the throat
- Hard, like the bony ribcage, the balls of the feet together form the chest and breast reflexes with the dome at the base being the diaphragm
- The fleshy insteps resemble the soft abdominal cavity
- The dense heel is solid like the bony pelvis.

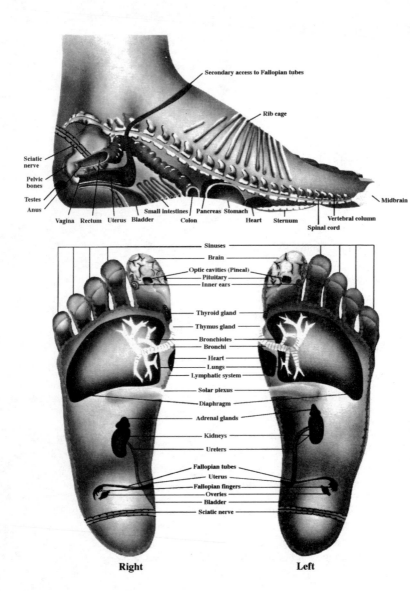

Figure 2 The reflection of bodily parts in miniature on the feet

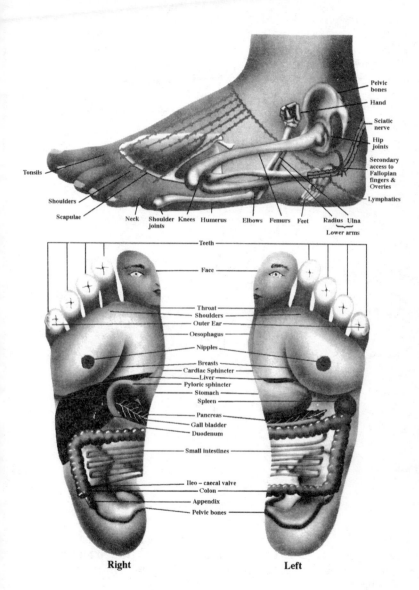

Right

Left

- The solid upper surfaces of both feet reflect the back of the body and carry the marks and characteristics of all that goes on 'behind the back' or the emotions that have been placed in the background
- Below each little toe, on the tops of the feet, the protruding bone matches the upper arm socket (Figure 3)
- Bony protrusions halfway down the outer edges of both feet correspond to the elbow joints (Figure 3)
- Both outer ankle-bones represent the sides of the hip-bones (Figure 3).

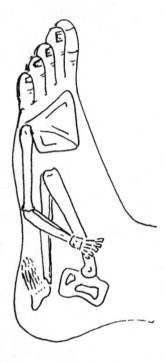

Figure 3   Limb reflexes on the sides of both feet

- All limb reflexes are represented by various bone formations on the outer edges of both feet (Figure 3). Limb reflexes are also present on the soles with the legs bent in front of the body in a sitting position (Figure 4)

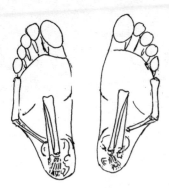

Figure 4 Sitting position on the soles of the feet

- Knobbly ridges of bone, from the joints on the medial edges of both big toes, along the inside surfaces of the feet, to beneath the inner ankle-bones, reflect the vertebrae in the spine (Figure 5)
- The right half of the spine is reflected along the inner edge of the right foot, and the left side of the spine along the inner edge of the left foot (Figure 5).

Visualisation of the position of the various bodily reflexes, as reflected directly onto the feet, simplifies the reflexology massage considerably.

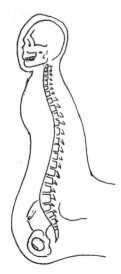

Figure 5 The spine reflexes

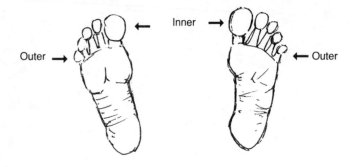

Figure 6 Inner and outer aspects of feet

For the purpose of this book, **inner edge** refers to reflexes on the **medial** aspect of the feet and toes, whilst **outer edge** specifies reflexes on the lateral parts (Figure 6).

❝ The feet are perfect microcosms of the body and carry the impressions of life. ❞

———— The effects of reflexology ————

After receiving reflexology recipients generally feel alert, rejuvenated and refreshed and at the same time relaxed and at ease. The feet tingle delightfully and the step is lighter.

With tension released, lively circulation within the relaxed blood vessels distributes nutrients and vital life-forces throughout, whilst accommodating more toxic, wasteful substances for easy elimination and detoxification. Expulsion of life-threatening substances is synonymous with letting go of menacing, worthless emotions that are potentially destructive.

Reflexology immediately dispenses with unwanted contents to remove all impediments to personal growth and self-development. Exoneration of emotional burdens lightens mind, body and soul, creating inner peace and homoeostasis.

Conditions are then ideal for natural, efficient functioning, physically, mentally, emotionally and spiritually. On the quantum level, the body's energy fields are totally regenerated and rejuvenated.

A simple explanation to those who know nothing about reflexology reassures the recipient about this trustworthy natural process and encourages them to let go.

❦ With an appropriate attitude aptitude can attain altitude. ❧

— Relief of common ailments — through the reflexology massage

Reflexology relieves common ailments by the subconscious release of emotional fears that traumatise, distort and distress the body. The relief of letting go eases mind, body and soul and places them back on track for a fulfilling, creative reality.

Healing occurs naturally when:

- the mind accepts and expresses individuality
- personal talents are realised and utilised
- there is understanding through unconditional love.

Recuperation occurs when there is:

- physical relief from distressing symptoms
- eradication of the emotion behind the dis-ease
- a change of mind to avoid re-occurrence
- inner harmony and peace
- an interest in getting better.

All this is facilitated, encouraged and made possible through reflexology, which encourages individuals to help themselves to a better way of life.

❦ Healing forces are within, not without. Therapies merely facilitate co-ordination of the mental and spiritual forces for inner harmony and peace. The body can and does heal itself. ❧

4

PREPARING FOR THE REFLEXOLOGY MASSAGE

To begin!

Reflexology is incredibly easy to learn since it is an inborn skill waiting to be alerted and utilised. Instinctive acts are frequently used to relieve discomfort. Many people intuitively:

- rub the skin to ease bumps and aching joints or muscles
- use saliva to soothe bites or stem minor blood flows
- scratch to relieve itching and irritability
- stroke an upset, grieving soul to reassure them
- massage the skin's surface to stimulate circulation or ease troubled, aching areas.

Reflexology is an instinctive knowledge guided by intuition, the only pre-requisite being an appreciation of life and all it stands for, so that the potential for leading an outstanding existence can be realised.

Reflexology is particularly beneficial when you are:

- stuck in a rut
- lacking direction
- feeling alone and misunderstood
- wondering what life is all about
- believing there is more to living
- questioning what the world is coming to.

This natural form of healing puts everything back into perspective, and creates a mind shift that makes the difference between 'having a life' and 'living a life'!

Ready to begin? Let's get started!

❝ Only by venturing into and exploring the unknown is the fullness and beauty of life appreciated. ❞

General preparation

Equipment required for reflexology consists mainly of standard household goods. Preparation of these prior to the massage is essential for the peaceful ambience necessary to administer relaxing reflexology.

- A bed, settee, reclining chair or massage couch, on which the recipient can lie and relax.
- Several pillows, with one to support the head and the remainder to wedge under the knees and legs for maximum comfort.
- Fresh, clean sheets in summer and blankets, duvets or quilts in winter to cover the recipient for modesty and to retain bodily heat which is often reduced as the body relaxes.
- Cushion, stool or chair for the administrator to sit on so that the recipient's feet are at eye level and at a manageable height
- A plastic bowl or foot bath for soaking the feet.
- A music centre, ideally with a repeat button, and some soothing tapes or compact discs to calm the nerves and enhance relaxation (see Appendix III).
- Optional extras are an aroma lamp and aromatherapy oils, or incense sticks that infiltrate the air with a subtle fragrance (see Appendix I).
- A beneficial accessory is an activated telephone answering machine to avoid interruption!
- Place a message on the door to prevent untimely intrusions.
- Although not essential, a dimmer switch reduces the glare of artificial lighting, particularly when dark, otherwise light soft-coloured candles, which in themselves are therapeutic.
- Attract bird life with seeds, and possibly invest in a fountain since bird song and running water add tranquillity.
- A container of powder near the administrator to facilitate the massage and reduce self-consciousness, especially when there is an unpleasant odour from extreme anxiety or the expulsion of toxic substances.
- Bach Flower Rescue Remedy drops for unexpected panic or shock and calcium tablets for possible cramp.

- Purified water in the fridge, with two glasses on a tray, for after the treatment, to assist in flushing out toxic substances
- Pastel colours soothe, whilst bright colours stimulate, so if possible choose furnishings with care, so that once the eyes are closed, and all environmental impressions are shut out, the recipient can drift into a blissful state of relaxation.

Create a peaceful setting in a subdued environment to invite total relaxation and escapism from the frenetic hustle and bustle of the outside world.

Now to begin.

Personal preparation

It is extremely rewarding to see amazing results so quickly, but it is important to remember that the administrator is only the conduit and facilitator who directs universal energies towards the recipient so that the healing process is accelerated. Healing comes from within and individuals heal themselves.

For the most beneficial massage:

- Gently rest the recipient's feet in the palms of your hands, in the most comfortable position for both (Figure 7)

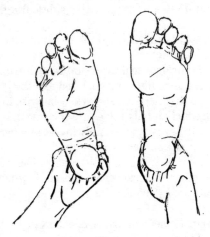

Figure 7 Resting the feet in both hands

- Take in three long, deep breaths, holding each breath for as long as possible ... then whilst exhaling feel the tension seep from your body as the muscles relax and create easiness throughout the whole. Repeat three times. Then continue to breathe naturally
- Consciously relax any particularly tense areas especially in your neck, shoulders, back and upper arms by concentrating on the taut parts and breathing into them in the same way as above
- Close your eyes and centre inwards by focusing attention and directing energies to your heart
- Clear your mind of all thoughts and be instinctively guided by intuition
- Tune into the recipient's needs to determine what the feet are 'saying'
- Do not try to please. Just be yourself
- Enjoy administering the massage
- Vary the pressure of the massage movements from being gentle but firm for physical ease to barely touching for personal enlightenment, to satisfy the needs of the mind, body and soul
- For particularly sensitive souls, visualise two beautiful pink bubbles, one around the body and the aura of yourself and the other around the recipient, to unconditionally allow each of you to enjoy your individual energies and space.

During and after the reflexology massage complete serenity, inner peace and a tremendous energy boost should be experienced not only by the recipient, but by the administrator as well.

❛ We have all bought a gift to the planet – ourselves – our uniqueness. ❜

❛ A smile shortens the distance between two people. ❜

—— Preparation of recipient ——

Before commencing a reflexology massage, briefly describe to the recipient:

- what reflexology is (page 3)
- how it works (page 19)
- possible experiences during and after the massage (pages 38 and 40)
- the reasons for any reactions (page 40)

- why it is advisable to drink plenty of purified water after the massage (page 41).

An explanation is generally appreciated whether or not the recipient has previously received this form of healing.

Anyone undergoing medical treatment should first advise the specialist of their intention to receive reflexology so that appropriate adjustments can be made in the dosages to accommodate improvements through acceleration of the healing process, which may be rapid. The best time for reflexology when receiving medication is one hour prior to the imminent dose. This is when the influence of drugs is minimal and the body is in its most vulnerable and receptive state.

Invite the recipient to soak their bare feet in a foot spa or plastic bowl for a few minutes:

- Use warm water in winter and cool water in summer
- Add a sprig of lavender or a drop of lavender aromatherapy oil for relaxation
- In summer a drop of peppermint aromatherapy oil cools and refreshes
- Provide a small clean towel for each recipient to dry the feet.

This is an ideal time to chat and explain reflexology. The recipient then lies on the bed, lazy-boy or couch in a comfortable position:

- Place one pillow beneath the head, if required, and several pillows under the knees and lower legs, to flatten and relax the spine.
- Cover with a light sheet in summer and a warm blanket or duvet in winter for modesty and to retain heat lost through relaxation
- Sit comfortably at the recipient's feet which should be placed at a convenient height for massage
- Prepare the self (page 30) and invite the recipient to also close the eyes and take in three long, deep breaths. Explain the breathing process beforehand.
- Shake powder into one hand, rub the hands together and then with both hands spread it gently over the feet and between the toes
- Lack of conversation during the massage allows the recipient to drift into the tranquil alpha state and reconnect with the inner self
- It is now time for the warm-up technique (page 46).

❻ Many feel a sense of nothingness and worthlessness, but within everyone is the ability to invent and create. Treat everyone, therefore, as the most precious person in the world. ❾

5
THE TECHNIQUE

Reflexology massage movements

An effective reflexology massage relies primarily on therapeutic touch and the personal approach, since any caress of the skin evokes an emotion either consciously or subconsciously. Reflexology values a sensitive application with unconditional acceptance since the administrator's feelings are immediately conveyed to the recipient.

Massage movements gently loosen and break down fixation with time to release mind, body and soul from being entrapped by belief systems that no longer apply.

Aggressive, threatening actions alert the recipient to recoil or lash out in self-defence, whereas acts of love and acceptance boost self-confidence and create a trusting environment to ease distress.

The soothing strokes of the reflexology:

- revitalise all bodily functions
- calm the nerves
- create inner harmony
- stimulate the circulatory and lymphatic systems
- strengthen the immune system
- pacify over-active glands and organs
- arouse sluggish bodily parts
- relax the muscles

- eliminate toxic substances
- relieve tension and distress
- lower high blood pressure
- increase low blood pressure
- ease aches and pains
- reduce swelling
- energise and rejuvenate mind, body and soul.

The need for touch increases during times of illness, distress or insecurity since, emotionally, the therapeutic touch of massage can:

- pacify
- induce confidence
- reassure
- free from distress
- create security
- increase acceptability.

Until recently the reflexology technique concentrated on the all-important physical and mechanical approach, but with the rapid shift in consciousness, it has expanded to keep pace with modern needs, making it one of the most all-encompassing therapies.

Staying tuned to the recipient needs helps determine the type of touch required, whether it should be firm or light. Physical people tend to prefer a more definite, harder technique initially but this modifies with increased personal awareness. Spiritual souls generally favour a more gentle, even non-physical approach, but there may be times when they need to be brought down to earth and grounded with a slightly firmer touch.

Three simple movements used on each reflex throughout the whole reflexology massage meet the ever-changing personal requirements through adjustments of pressure. These variations can differ from one part of the foot to another and from treatment to treatment but they do allow fluctuating physical and emotional requirements of individuals to be balanced.

Intuition provides guidance regarding the amount of pressure needed since it may vary considerably from the two extremes of being firm to having no physical contact during a single massage.

Practise the following techniques on the hand first, to gain confidence.

The caterpillar movement

Place the tips of both thumbs lightly on the skin's surface and then gently drop the thumbs so that their pads rest lightly on the skin. Rock the thumbs back onto their tips then once again ease them back down onto their pads. Continue to 'walk' the thumbs *forwards* in this manner (Figure 8).

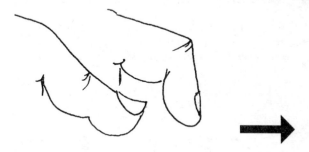

Figure 8 The caterpillar movement

The rotation action

Gently place the tips of both thumbs or, if preferred, fingers onto the reflex points and without moving the digits create a vibration by slightly gyrating the digits on both points of contact. If resistance is felt or the reflex feels drained of energy, lightly press onto the reflexes and hold the pressure momentarily. Very slowly ease off whilst rotating the digits at the same time (Figure 9).

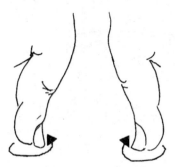

Figure 9 Rotation movement

Use either or both of the above techniques on each reflex first to:

- relax muscular tension
- ease physical distress
- calm the nerves
- relieve aches, pains and so on.

The stroking or milking movement

Place the thumbs or fingers firmly but lightly on the reflexes and reassuringly stroke the skin's surface in either long, soothing sweeps or shorter movements whilst applying slight pressure (Figure 10).

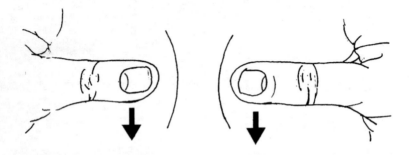

Figure 10 Stroking or milking movement

The stroking or milking movement can also be done individually on each reflex, thumb over thumb or finger over finger (Figure 11).

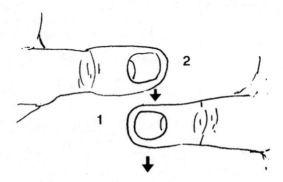

Figure 11 Milking movement – thumb over thumb

The stroking or milking movement is applied to each reflex after the caterpillar or rotation massage to:

- soothe the emotions
- create inner harmony and ease
- eliminate threatening feelings.

The feather or healing movement

This is similar to the stroking or milking action, but this time the skin's surface is caressed with the lightest of touches, or without touching at all!

Use this gentle technique to:

- reassure and reconnect with the true self at soul level.

   ❛ Health and healing are natural when in touch with the soul. ❜

The effects of the massage movements

For best results, massage every reflex in both feet with each movement, giving the greatest attention to the brain, spinal, solar plexus and endocrine gland reflexes. Two or more hours may be required initially to complete a full massage but, with confidence and practice, this can be reduced to an hour.

Detailed techniques for the various parts of the feet are described in the relevant section of the book. Each movement during reflexology massage:

- *activates* by toning and strengthening especially sluggish, hypo-active areas that require stimulation
- *pacifies* by calming and soothing particularly nervous, hyperactive parts.

Whether giving reflexology for the maintenance of health or for a specific dis-ease always massage both feet thoroughly, concentrating on congested, swollen areas or parts that lack vibrancy. These are easily detected on the skin's surface through:

- resistance or hardness due to fear, anxiety or vulnerability
- magnetism from a need for energy and rejuvenation
- flatness, unresponsiveness or dullness from feeling drained and exhausted.

On these unnatural reflexes:

- lightly rest a digit on the spot to re-energise, or
- apply gentle pressure and slowly release until there is minimal contact, or
- increase the rotation technique to reawaken and stimulate the reflex.

Respect individual belief systems to know intuitively what is best for all concerned. Results may be amazing even after one treatment but by not taking the credit for the healing there should be no loss of confidence when there is no apparent reaction. The outcome of treatments may be affected by the recipient's choice to improve or otherwise. The process of healing can be blocked or slowed down when the recipient receives greater sympathy and attention during illness and dis-ease. It is then not in their interest to get better if they usually feel insignificant.

The less effort and personal will imposed during reflexology, the better the results. Instinctive actions and reactions ensure the best possible outcome for all concerned.

❢ It's not **what** is done, but the love with which it is administered that determines effectiveness! ❧

Sensations experienced during the reflexology massage

During the exquisite alpha level of consciousness into which the recipient drifts during reflexology massage, there is an acute awareness of surrounding noise and activity but any concern is overridden by a pleasant detachment that dispenses with the need to be involved. In this way the recipient never loses conscious control, despite appearing to be in a deep sleep.

The variety of sensations experienced during a reflexology massage are very individual and it is impossible to determine a recipient's reaction.

Extreme tenderness indicates a high level of tension whilst excessive sensitivity acts as an alarm that alerts the whole to be defensive due to fear or insecurity.

An explanation of possible reactions provides insight into why certain feelings are experienced:

- Heat loss as the body relaxes and lets off steam, particularly when uptight
- A sinking feeling with relaxation
- Floating as burdens dissipate and take a weight off the whole
- Twitching and jerking of previously deprived, tense areas with the penetration and surge of energy and vitality
- Plucking hand movements due to frustration or uncertainty in handling situations
- 'Pins and needles' sensation or numbness in the hands from a subconscious dread of handling circumstances
- Snoring releases deeply suppressed emotions kept close to the chest, common particularly in the alpha state
- Beautiful colours, ranging from subdued, subtle hues to exceptionally bright ones, even with the eyes closed.

Less common reactions are:

- Out-of-body experiences as the soul temporarily leaves the body for a different point of view
- Recall of previous life situations
- Feeling a murky lining of emotional trash being pulled out of the body like a piece of material to be finally dispensed with
- Singing out loud with songs such as 'Please release me'.

Whatever happens, no matter how peculiar or unexpected, reactions are perfect for all concerned.

During reflexology massage breathing becomes shallow and almost undetectable so, at the end of the massage, ask the recipient to take three deep breaths to bring themselves out of this incredibly relaxed state. There may be a reluctance to leave such bliss, so allow time.

Ideally, if the recipient is in a bed and can roll over to sleep, then even greater benefit can be derived from the reflexology massage. They will wake up feeling fantastic!

> ‘Natural therapies evoke natural responses, for enrichment of mind, body and soul.’

—— After-effects of reflexology ——

As a revitalising and rejuvenating therapy, the most common reaction to reflexology is renewed enthusiasm and vitality for life. Many find that they:

- think more clearly
- have increased tolerance
- can concentrate better
- feel more at ease with themselves and others
- have greater confidence
- are able to achieve more
- have abundant energy
- sleep increasingly soundly and awake refreshed
- dream more often for personal guidance and understanding
- have greater empathy for bodily and soul needs
- are reluctant to abuse mind, body or soul
- have a clearer concept of the soul's purpose
- find a direction filling the whole with renewed enthusiasm
- enjoy the quality of life to the full.

A total personality change from being a disgruntled, aggressive, obstinate grouch to being an affable, patient and accommodating soul occurs frequently.

For change to take place, a thorough spring clean is required to remove the old and make way for the new. Reflexology massage accelerates this purification process. Although initially disturbing, exhausting or disruptive, once completed there is a fantastic feeling of liberation and release.

Reflexology works with and not against the manifestations of illness, completing the cycle of dis-ease, thoroughly eliminating all toxic substances. Any of the following are excellent signs that the body is helping itself to better health.

- A headache from past hurts coming to a head for final eradication
- High temperatures to let off steam and eliminate heated emotions
- Increased perspiration to flush out old fears
- Runny eyes to release unshed tears and wash away hurtful sights
- A cold or a runny nose to clean out all past irritants

- Skin rashes or eruptions to allow irrational, boiling emotions under the skin to surface and escape
- Females may experience a more virulent vaginal discharge to dismiss frustrating female issues
- Increased urination to provide relief from inappropriate aspects of relationships
- Frequent, easier defecation to let go of the wasteful remnants of life's processes
- Temporary diarrhoea to dispense with unnecessary nonsense and unreasonable pressure
- Vivid recall of dreams to help comprehension of life events.

Encourage the recipient to drink plenty of purified water after a reflexology massage to assist the flushing-through process and to hasten the release of inhibiting thoughts and emotions that make life heavy going.

Explain to the recipient the reasons for possible reactions so that they are aware of what to expect and why.

❛ Life can be understood backwards but must be lived forwards! ❜

— **Unusual but possible reactions** —

Natural stimulants evoke natural responses, so it is impossible to cause harm with the light, but firm, movements used in reflexology.

However, life continually provides opportunities to test inner strength to prove the ability to cope with challenging situations as part of the growth experience, and it is possible that during reflexology a perceivably alarming reaction **may** appear. If so, remain calm and be intuitively guided to know what to do. Remember that no one is given more than they can cope with.

As a non-invasive, natural therapy, reflexology causes dormant conditions to come to a head. If rapid, this may be alarming and appear to be an adverse reaction – it is, in fact, an excellent sign that the healing process has been activated.

Palpitations, hyperventilation or panic may occur from a subconscious arousal of heart-wrenching emotions that require immediate release. Stay calm! Whenever a response causes concern, always pacify by:

- immediately placing the digits on the solar plexus reflexes (page 92)
- asking the recipient to take in deep, long breaths and relax
- reassure the recipient that the reaction is temporary
- if available, administer Bach Flower Rescue Remedy to provide further reassurance.

The recipient should begin to feel more tranquil immediately, but be patient if it takes longer.

Continue with the massage once the recipient has settled down. On completion, encourage them to drink more purified water than usual to flush out any extra toxins and suggest they return as soon as possible for a further massage to continue balancing out the whole.

These reactions are not common, but it is important to be aware of them so that appropriate action can be taken.

❜ Each individual is completely responsible for personal thoughts, actions and reactions. ❜

——— First-aid reflexology ———

Ideally, a complete massage on both feet is required for total balance of mind, body and soul. Occasionally, however, insufficient time will dictate a 'quick massage', which is better than nothing. For this:

- massage all toes thoroughly (page 58)
- soothe the spinal reflexes (page 66)
- pacify the solar plexus reflexes (page 92)
- balance the energy centres (page 128)
- always finish with an overall massage of both feet, using stroking movements towards the recipient's body. In this way, energies are flushed through to benefit the mind, body and soul.

To ease extreme discomfort in a particular part of the body:

- massage the distressed reflex(es) (see index)
- then calm the solar plexus reflexes (page 92)
- continue with the whole procedure or the 'quick massage' above.

6

THE REFLEXOLOGY MASSAGE

The sequence

Begin reflexology massage with a general massage, known as the warm-up (page 46). The order of reflexology massage is then as follows:

- The **toes** (page 58) with the *brain* and *sensory reflexes* to:
  – ease the mind
  – soothe the emotions
  – alert the senses.
- The knobbly **ridge of bone** along the inside edges of both feet reflecting the *spine reflexes* (page 65) and the *solar plexus reflexes* (page 92) in the hollows beneath the balls of the feet to:
  – calm the nerves
  – relax the musculature
  – release tension
  – improve circulation
  – enhance the natural functioning of all bodily systems.
- The **toe necks** (page 75) to:
  – ease neck and throat tension
  – facilitate the exchange of natural life-forces, e.g. air
  – open the avenues of expression, e.g. speech.
- The **balls** (page 85) of the feet containing the *chest, breast, heart* and *upper arm reflexes* to:
  – boost self-esteem and self-worth
  – provide space for personal feelings
  – get retained emotions off the chest
  – ease snoring and respiratory tension.

- The **insteps** (page 106) which reflect the bulk of the *digestive tract*, as well as most of the *urinary tract reflexes* to:
  - harmonise the digestive process
  - ease break down, assimilation and absorption of life
  - purify the whole body
  - form and maintain fulfilling relationships
  - relieve abdominal discomfort.
- *Pelvic* and *leg reflexes* in the **heels** (page 127) to:
  - revitalise body, mind and soul with renewed energy and enthusiasm for lively participation in the journey through life
  - enhance personal growth and development
  - increase personal security
  - relieve skeletal and muscular tension.
- Finally, the finale (page 133) involves general manipulation to:
  - release any remaining tension
  - loosen the tight grip on life
  - enhance relaxation
  - increase flexibility for overall well-being.

  ❛ The cycles of nature defy a linear approach to life. ❜

— General observations of the feet —

Vibrant, healthy feet with a flesh-coloured hue are pliable, relaxed and able to adapt and fit into life's situations with ease. Tension alarms and rigidifies the feet, creating resistance. Hard skin builds up in areas of perceived vulnerability to protect or conceal true emotions. Callouses, corns and extra skin signify subconscious thoughts, fears and anxiety, with their position on the foot pinpointing the exact feeling.

Skin texture should be naturally firm but supple and reveals the degree of vibrancy and the energy level.

- Flaccid skin gives in too easily under pressure due to temporary lack of substance
- Skin toughness during perceivably difficult phases creates a barrier against being hurt or through an act of defiance
- Continual friction rubs the skin up the wrong way, making it shine, rough or blister
- During transition periods the skin peels to let go of the old and make way for the new.

Colouring of skin reveals consistently changing moods and feelings. Many colours may be present on the feet at any one time and these alter perpetually with shifting emotions.

- When tired and exhausted, feet are drained of colour and look white
- Anger and frustration create heated emotions that inflame the mind, turning the face and feet red
- Brown feet reveal feelings of being 'browned off' or act as a cover up
- Yellow in the feet displays extreme annoyance
- Tinges of green reveal moments of envy
- Emotional hurt causes the skin to turn black and blue from feeling battered. The depth of colour indicates the degree of hurt and bruised sentiment.

The angle of feet is significant:

- in a standing or sitting position, feet point in the direction of interest or indicate the overriding thought that holds the greatest attention. This is done either with confident open-mindedness or self-centred uncertainty.
- in the prone position feet should stand upright, but are:
  - drawn to the person's right when temporarily pulled back into the past, or
  - give preference to the left side of the body when looking ahead and projecting into the future.
- when walking:
  - parallel feet are on track
  - open feet try to please and accommodate others
  - pigeon-toed feet temporarily lack confidence and cut off the outside world.

The right foot carries the marks of past experiences whilst the left foot is more concerned with present thoughts and feelings. Positive, masculine energies rebound mainly in the right foot, whereas the left foot gives preference to the negative female energies, although each cell has both male/female and positive/negative energies.

‘Feet are our autobiographies.’

Footnote: *The Language of the Feet*, also written by Chris Stormer and published by Hodder and Stoughton, provides deeper insight into the ever-changing and fascinating characteristics of the feet. With life constantly changing and people striving to progress, this understanding makes it easier to tune into the recipient's individual needs, which differ from massage to massage.

The warm-up

General loosening-up techniques for initial relaxation

The caressing movements of the warm-up:

- encourage initial relaxation
- form a trusting relationship
- provide an ideal opportunity to gauge recipient's needs.

Adapt the following techniques to suit the recipient's needs:

Step 1

- Gently stroke the top of the right foot, several times, hand over hand, towards the self, and then stroke the sole of the right foot with the backs of the hands (Figure 12).
- Repeat on the left foot.

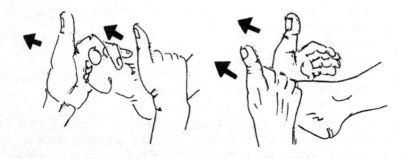

Figure 12 Stroking, hand over hand

Step 2

- Place the tips of all fingers on top of the toes on the right foot.
- With tiny circular movements, massage with all fingers moving from the toes up to the ankle (Figure 13).

- Separate the hands at the ankles to thoroughly massage either side of the right heel, especially around the ankle-bone.
- Repeat on the left foot.

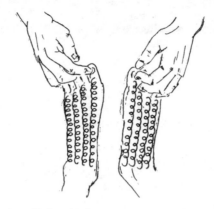

Figure 13 Massaging with tiny circular movements

Step 3

- The recipient must lie flat for this next movement, known as the *achilles pull* (Figure 14).
- Rest the right heel in the palm of the stronger hand, and then align the other hand with the top of the right foot.
- Gently, but firmly, draw the right heel towards yourself, to extend the right leg, until a slight resistance is felt.

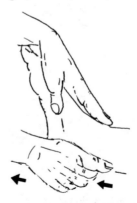

Figure 14 Achilles pull

Step 4

- Ease the pull and keeping both hands in position, bend the foot down, with the palm of the hand on top, to extend the upper surface of the foot (Figure 15).
- Repeat Steps 3 and 4 alternately at least three times before manipulating the left foot.

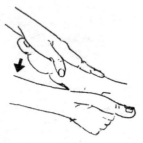

Figure 15 Achilles stretch

The techniques in Steps 3 and 4 are exceptionally good for headaches, neck and back problems since they extend the spine and pressure on entrapped, impinged nerves is lessened.

Step 5

- With the third fingers massage around the right ankle-bones. Initially apply a firm but gentle pressure, using circular movements, and then gradually ease off until there is little or no contact with the skin's surface (Figure 16).
- All digits can be used to massage.

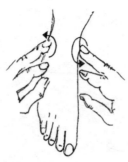

Figure 16 Massaging the ankles

- Repeat on the left ankle.
- Massage well to facilitate movement through life by increasing flexibility in the hip joints.

Step 6

- Place the mounds at the bases of both thumbs in the hollows either side of the right ankle bones so that they rest comfortably.
- Keeping contact move one hand up and one hand down to manipulate the whole of the right foot from side to side (Figure 17).
- With practice, this movement can be speeded up to loosen any stiffness.
- Repeat on the left foot.

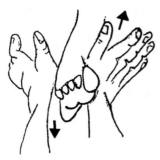
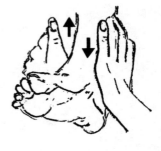

Figure 17 Foot shake

Step 7

- Make a fist with the left hand and place towards the outer edge of the right sole, immediately under the necks of the toes.

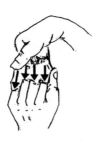
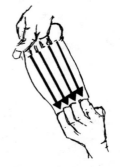

Figure 18 Knuckle down massage

- Now use the right hand to gently support the toes, whilst stroking the soles, from top to bottom, with the flat of the left knuckle (Figure 18).
- Massage in strips from the outer to the inner edge of the right foot.
- Repeat on the left foot, reversing the role of the hands.

Step 8

- Use the heel on the palm of the right hand to gently stroke the arch of the right instep, towards the recipient, applying slight pressure to the bony ridge (Figure 19).
- Repeat several times and then stroke the left arch with the heel of the palm on the left hand.

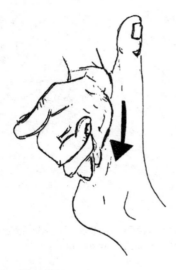

Figure 19 Stroking the arch

Stroke both feet, from toes to ankles, then proceed to the massage of the toes.

❛ Live well for today,
For yesterday is a dream,
And tomorrow a vision.

But today well lived
Makes every yesterday a dream of happiness,
And every tomorrow a vision of hope. ❜

7

THE TOES

All toes reflect the head, which, via the brain, consciously, subconsciously and unconsciously determines the condition and health of mind, body and soul (Figure 20).

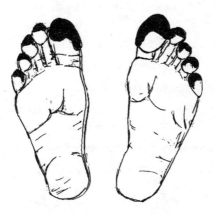

Figure 20 The brain reflexes on the toes

Nerve fibres infiltrate the whole body and so the spinal cord reflexes are massaged after the toes to facilitate the relay of messages to and from the brain (Figure 21).

❛ Life is an adventure of the mind, that makes the impossible possible. ❜

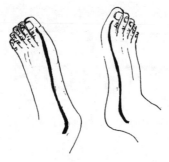

Figure 21 The spinal cord and vertebral reflexes

—— Position of the toe reflexes ——

Toe nails represent the skull bone, at the back of head.

Toe pads mirror the face with the right side of the face on the right toe pad and the left side of the face on the left toe pad.

Upper part of toe pads reflect brain and sinuses.

Outer border of toes portray the sides of the head and ear reflexes.

Central mound of toe pads reflect eyes.

Inner edge of toes centre: nose and pituitary gland reflexes;
        lower: mouth, teeth and gum.

Bottom rim of toe pads denote the jaw reflexes.

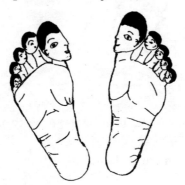

Figure 22 The face reflexes on all toes

Impact of tension on the toe reflexes

Pressure on the cranium prevents the overall distribution of essential life-forces to the brain cells, depriving them of the opportunity to function to their maximum potential. This can result in:

- lack of concentration
- inability to think clearly
- irritability and impatience
- pain and aching in the head
- pressure on the mind, leaving no space for thought
- baldness as hair follicles become entrapped
- aggravation of the senses, distorting, amplifying, exaggerating and misconstruing perceptions.

If accompanied by anger and frustration, infection may occur, resulting in:

- inflammation of the meninges, the brain's covering, arising from frustration in the belief that personal concepts and ideas need to be concealed or protected.

Influence of reflexology on the toes

Massage of the toes:

- clears the mind
- improves concentration
- increases tolerance
- raises the level of consciousness
- intensifies perception and the senses, particularly intuition
- encourages overall well-being and general health.

The relationship of all toes, especially the big toes, to the nervous system means that massage of the toes can:

- calm the nerves
- clarify and strengthen the relationship between the brain and the rest of the body

- heighten natural sensitivity
- co-ordinate muscular control
- encourage appropriate physical, intellectual, emotional and spiritual communication
- create an environment of inner harmony and ease
- evoke suitable thoughts and feelings
- incite healthy actions and reactions
- enhance internal and external relationships.

Outcome of reflexology on individual toes

Each pair of toes reflects specific aspects of the multi-talented, expansive mind, the functioning of which can be developed further through the reflexology massage.

Big toe stimulates intellect, intuition and clarity of thought.

Second toe boosts perceptions of self-worth and self-esteem.

Third toe encourages and inspires ideas to be put into practice.

Fourth toe enhances communication and personal relationships.

Little toe expands and frees the mind from inhibiting belief systems. Innovative ideas can then challenge and replace outdated and limiting thought patterns.

Effect of reflexology on specific toe reflexes

Massage of specific parts of the toe pads directly effects the corresponding part as well as the whole body.

The toe pads

Toe pads reflect the face and its features. Through reflexology it is possible to:

- boost self-confidence
- ease confrontation

- assist in facing life situations
- enhance individual identity.

The tips of the toe pads

The tips of the toes reflect the brain and sinus reflexes. Massage these to:

- activate brain activity
- improve intellect and intuition
- prolong concentration
- alter thought patterns for a healthy state of mind, body and soul
- take a weight off the mind
- provide space to think and play around with ideas.

The centre of the toe pads

The mounds in the centres of the toe pads contain the eye reflexes which reflect the accuracy with which light waves are focused into meaningful shapes for:

- accurate interpretation of environmental conditions
- clear vision
- insight and intuition.

The control of all cycles throughout mind, body and soul is the natural function of the pineal gland, which relies on the vibrant health of the eyes. Massage the central portion of all toe pads to:

- sharpen vision
- ease eye strain
- improve intuition
- enlighten mind, body and soul
- harmonise natural cycles, particularly the menstrual cycle in women and mood swings.

The outer aspect of the toes – little toe side

On the outer joints of all toes are the ear reflexes which reflect the precision with which sound waves are transformed into comprehensive signals. Through direction, guidance and balance from the inner voice, personal growth and development are enhanced. Stimulate these reflexes to:

- heighten listening abilities
- improve balance
- ease hearing disorders
- clarify the meaning of sounds
- facilitate understanding and accurate interpretation.

The inner edge of the toes – big toe side

Along the inside edges over the joints, particularly of the big toe, are the midbrain reflexes (Figure 23) that balance muscular co-ordination and contain the cardiac and respiratory centres.

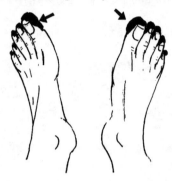

Figure 23 Midbrain reflexes

The reflexes of the pituitary gland, the master endocrine gland, are also found here (Figure 24). They reflect the control of all hormonal activity for inner emotional harmony and inner peace.

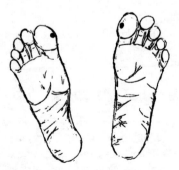

Figure 24 Pituitary gland reflexes

The nose reflexes overlap the two above reflexes and reveal effective detection of the evocative sense of smell. This sense heightens with increased acceptance and recognition of the self.

Massage these bony protuberances to:

- improve muscular co-ordination
- enhance the sense of smell
- boost personal recognition
- create inner peace and harmony
- balance emotions
- calm nerves
- refine inner communication.

The lower part of the toe pad

Immediately below the nose reflexes are the reflexes of the mouth. This cavity facilitates the two-way exchange and communication of energies between the internal and external worlds for meaningful, beneficial relationships.

Along the lower edge of the toe pad is the reflex of the jaw, which acts as a firm, mobile base for thoughts and perceptions, and provides the strength and mobility to express ideas.

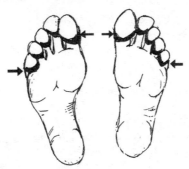

Figure 25 Jaw reflexes

Massage the lower toe pad to:

- facilitate speech
- ease decision making
- increase self-confidence
- feel secure with personal concepts.

The upper surface of the toes

Toe nails reflect the cranium bone which shields the brain from harm or damage and protects or guards individual intellect and ideas from perceived criticism or mockery. Corns on top of the toes provide extra covering against others stamping and treading on the toes and personal concepts.

Massage of the upper toe surfaces:

- strengthens belief in personal concepts
- provides a firm backing to ideas
- opens the mind to every point of view.

— Reflexology massage of the toes —

The toes' direct relationship to the nervous system encourages physical, mental, emotional and spiritual peace and harmony. Always thoroughly massage all the toe reflexes first to:

- relax and balance mind, body and soul
- make space for rejuvenation and restoration by easing nervous tension
- encourage the natural functioning of all bodily parts, consciously, unconsciously and subconsciously.

Step 1

- Gently place the ends of all fingertips on top of all little toes (Figure 26).
- Slowly apply slight pressure for a few seconds, and then gradually ease off until the fingertips just rest on or hover immediately above the skin's surface.

Vibrancy or warmth felt between the fingers and toes is activated energy that revitalises both recipient and administrator.

Step 2

- Remove all fingers and gently place the ends of the third fingers on the tips of the big toes (Figure 27).

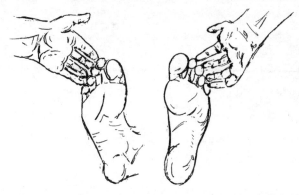

Figure 26 Fingertips on top of toes

- Again, apply slight pressure for a few seconds and then slowly ease off until the fingertips rest on or hover immediately above the big toes.

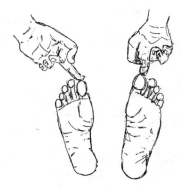

Figure 27 Third fingers on big toes

Step 3

- Place the tips of the thumbs or third fingers onto the outer edges over the little toes (Figure 28).
- Slowly apply slight pressure to these points for a few seconds and then, without moving the digits, gently rotate. (See caterpillar and rotation movements on page 35).
- Use this technique to progress along the top of all toes, finishing on the inner edge of the big toe.

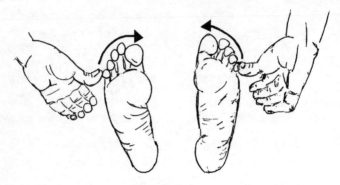

Figure 28 Massaging the tips of the toes

Step 4

- Repeat Step 3 but this time place both thumbs over the toe pads on the little toes and gently massage, with the third fingers placed directly opposite on top of the toes.
- The dual use of the digits can substantially increase the energy flow so if initially it proves too intense, keep the thumbs in position and remove the third fingers.

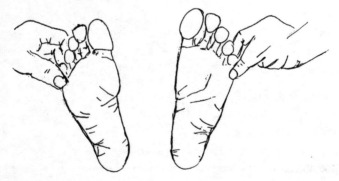

Figure 29 Massaging with the thumbs and third fingers

Step 5

- Continue to repeat this movement, each time moving fractionally further down the toe pads, until all pads have been thoroughly massaged. Spend time, especially on the big toes.

Step 6

- Concentrate on massaging the strips along the bases of the toe pads since these are the jaw reflexes and are often exceptionally tense.

Step 7

- Place the thumb pads on the outer tips of the little toes and soothingly but firmly stroke the outside edges of the little toe pads from top to bottom.
- The milking movement clears the lymphatic reflexes and, in so doing calms and reassures the mind. (See milking movement on page 36).

Step 8

- Repeat Step 7, each time moving the digits fractionally along the toe pads of both little toes (Figure 30).
- Stroke in strips from top to bottom until the whole pad has been milked.

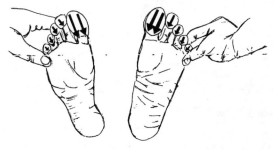

Figure 30 Milking the little toes

Step 9

- Repeat steps 7 and 8 but this time on the fourth toe, then the third toe and so on, finishing on the big toes.

Step 10

- Feather stroke (page 36) the right little toe pad, then the fourth, third, second and big toe until all toe pads on the right foot have been soothed.
- Repeat on the left toe pads in the same sequence, starting on the left little toe and ending on the left big toe.

This light movement lifts a weight off the mind, creates space to think clearly, raises the level of consciousness, soothes emotions and re-establishes contact at soul level.

Step 11

- Lightly place the thumbs or third fingers on the inner joints of the big toes, over the nose and pituitary gland reflexes (Figure 31).
- Gradually apply gentle pressure, whilst rotating the digits.
- Ease the pressure and then rest the third fingers on the reflexes for a few seconds.
- Visualise the colour violet to enhance the effect.

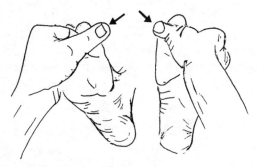

Figure 31 Massaging pituitary gland and nose reflexes

Massaging these reflexes:

- calms the emotions
- creates inner harmony
- boosts self-esteem and self-worth
- balances the secretion of hormones.

Step 12

- Now gently place the thumbs on the centres of both little toe pads, with the third fingers situated directly opposite on top of the little toes (Figure 32).
- Lightly squeeze the two digits together by applying slight pressure. When resistance is felt, hold for a few seconds, then slowly rotate the thumbs. Gradually ease the compression until both digits barely touch skin. Visualise the colour indigo whilst doing this to intensify the effect.

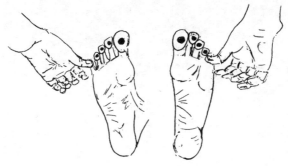

Figure 32 Massaging eye and pineal gland reflexes

● Now place both third fingers on the central portion of the fourth toes and repeat the massage. Then onto the third toes, second toes and finally the big toes.

Massaging the eye reflexes, especially the main reflexes on the big toes:

● expands intuitive perceptions
● clarifies and sharpens vision
● encourages maximum optical functioning.

Hormonal secretions from the pineal gland rely on healthy optic conditions since light transmission into the body through the eye determines the efficient functioning of this gland that controls all natural cycles. Stimulating this reflex:

● naturalises the menstrual cycle
● stabilises mood swings
● enhances intuition.

Step 13

● Place the thumbs on the inner joints and the third fingers on the outer joints of both little toes (Figure 33).
● Massage the sides of each toe, starting on the little toes and finishing on both edges of the big toes.
● Gently squeeze the digits together to apply slight pressure for a while. Then milk the sides of the toes from top to bottom, with minimal compression between the digits.
● Repeat on the fourth toes and then all toes, finishing on the big toes. Massage the big toes particularly well since they contain the main head, brain and sensory reflexes.

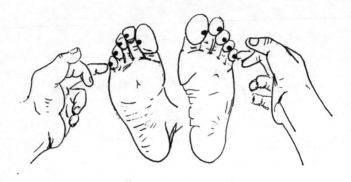

Figure 33 Massaging ear reflexes

The outer edges of each toe reflect nerves, muscle, skin, bone, circulatory and lymphatic vessels on the sides of the face, temple, ear and jaw.

The inner surfaces mirror the inside of the head, brain, pituitary gland, midbrain and cervical vertebrae including the nerves, muscle, skin, bone, circulatory and lymphatic vessels in those areas.

Step 14

- Place four fingers on the outer edges of both little toes and move them in unison to 'walk' them over the tops of the toes, to finish on the inner edges of the big toes (Figure 34).
- Repeat two to three times.

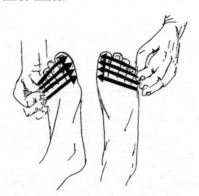

Figure 34 Walking the fingers over the tops of the toes

Step 15

- Now place the third fingers onto the tips of both little toes (Figure 35). Rest them for a few seconds then move them onto the joints of the little toes.
- Stay a while before finally resting them on the bases of both little toes for a while.
- Repeat on the fourth toes, the third toes, the second toes and lastly the big toes.

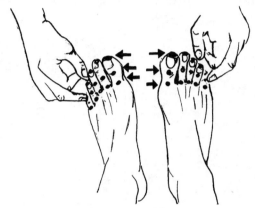

Figure 35   The three positions on the tops of the toes

These movements:

- increase energy flow to the brain
- clear mental congestion
- ease cranial pressure
- relax the neck muscles
- improve circulation between the brain and the rest of the body.

The spinal cord reflexes (see page 66) are massaged at this stage, to soothe and stimulate the nerves that infiltrate the rest of the body from the spine.

Massage of the spinal reflexes:

- facilitates the relay of nervous messages between the brain and the rest of the body
- increases and alerts each cell's awareness of the state and condition of the rest of the body

- improves the functioning of every body part for optimum efficiency and effectiveness.

Step 16

- Place the thumbs or fingers on the inner joints of both big toes and gently massage the length of the bony ridges that border the central portion of both feet ending at the lower edge of the inner ankles (immediately above the inner fleshy insteps).
- Repeat the massage two to three times.

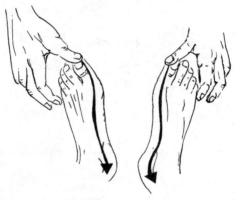

Figure 36 Massage of the spinal reflexes

These bones reflect the vertebral column which contains the spinal cord.

Step 17

- Milk the spinal reflexes, thumb over thumb or finger over finger, with small, repetitive soothing strokes towards the recipient, first up the right spinal reflex, from toe to ankle, and then along the left spinal reflex.
- Repeat several times to remove congested emotions.

Step 18

- Feather stroke both spinal reflexes with two fingers or both thumbs, in the same way as Step 17, but with an exceptionally light touch.
- Repeat a few times to soothe the nerves.

Step 19

Finally, the Metamorphic technique liberates past fears and anxieties, especially those experienced whilst in the womb since:

- the tips of the big toes represent the point of conception
- the spinal reflexes reflect the time in the womb
- the ankle represents the time of birth.

- Lightly place the tips of the third fingers on the top of both big toes and keep them still for a few seconds.
- Then, barely touching the skin's surface, slide the fingers slowly over both spinal reflexes, under the inner ankles finishing at the back of these bony protrusions.
- Remain here for a few seconds before repeating the stroking movement two to three times.
- A circular movement can also be used in conjunction with the above.

Bony vertebrae protect the fragile spinal cord and nerve fibres from harm and provide solid support and backing to body, mind and soul. The condition of the insteps reflect the strength of the spinal cord.

- Babies lack insteps due to total dependence on the support of others. Increased confidence of standing on their own two feet develops the insteps later.
- Throughout life the instep should remain stable and supportive but may collapse under pressure or at times of emotional strain, resulting in temporary flat feet.
- At times when extra support and backing are required the insteps overextend which increases the arch in an attempt to provide added support.

Stroke both feet before moving onto massage of the toe necks which follows on page 75.

❝ The wealth of knowledge gained through life's experiences can never be the same for two people who will respond according to their individual backgrounds. ❞

— Natural characteristics of the toes —

Healthy toes stand supply upright with fully exposed, firm, pliable pads of fleshy, vibrant hue.

——— Altered states of the toes ———

Thought patterns have direct impact on toe characteristics:

- The stature of toes determines the degree of confidence in standing up and facing the world with personal concepts and ideals.
- Pliant, flexible toes share individual ideas and concepts with ease.
- The degree of rigidity reflects the extent of personal insecurity and uncertainty.
- Toes bend and bow when:
  - succumbing to alien belief systems
  - lacking faith in own concepts
  - charging ahead and going head first regardless of the consequences.
- Misshapen toes try to accommodate unsuitable belief systems.
- Boxed toes contain personal concepts for fear of rejection or ridicule.
- Toe pads that lean or turn to the right of the body are influenced by the past, whilst those that turn to the left constantly look ahead into the future.
- The colouring of the toes reveals the emotional aspect of thought patterns:
  Red – frustrated, angry thoughts.
  White – too exhausted and drained to think.
  Yellow – fed up with type of mental activity.
  Black or *blue* – hurt notions.
  Green – envious or sick at the thought of present situation.
- Hard skin conceals, covers up or protects unique perceptions.
- Corns prevent ideas from being trampled upon.

——— Nervous disorders ———

All ailments are a form of nervous disorder since the health of the body reflects the state of mind. Happiness, inner calm and relaxation ease the musculature allowing the cells to function effectively and efficiently for the benefit of mind, body and soul.

Dis-ease displays, uneasiness, unhappiness and frustration, with life 'getting on the nerves'. A variety of specific symptoms reveal specific thought patterns and the type of emotion causing internal havoc and physical unrest.

Tension restricts and reduces the amount of blood flow and deprives the brain and nerve cells of essential life-forces. Pressure restricts the amount of space available for clear thought and efficient functioning. Feeling out of control, pressurised, anxious and unable to cope are a few of the possible manifestations.

When under strain, nervous impulses and messages conveyed along the finely tuned, highly sensitive nerve fibres can be distorted or traumatised by threatening thought patterns resulting in:

● Pain from emotional hurt
● Aching and longing for love and recognition
● Tension from extreme anger, frustration, fear and anxiety
● Nervousness from extreme uncertainty and inner havoc
● Infections, inflammations and high temperatures as outlets for contained festering thoughts, heated emotions or inflamed feelings surfacing for final release
● Convulsions from fits of rage that distort the brain waves and throw brain activity off course
● Excessive irritability with 'nerves on edge' from extreme intolerance and impatience of situations and/or people that threaten personal concepts. Often from the perceived need for perfection. Natural irritability prevents threatening substances from entering the body and is essential for survival
● Increased sensitivity from forces perceivably stronger, greater and more threatening than personal resistance. Natural sensitivity protects the whole from the adverse aspects of life.

Reflexology effectively dissipates all of the above by:

● opening the mind
● calming nerves
● boosting self-worth
● increasing the level of tolerance.

Specific nervous disorders eased through reflexology

For any disorder, a complete reflexology massage is required with the greatest emphasis being on:

- nervous system and solar plexus reflexes to calm the mind and relieve pain, fear and anxiety
- endocrine gland reflexes to soothe the emotions and create inner harmony
- affected gland or organ reflexes to relax the distressed area and ease the symptoms of dis-ease.

The following also includes aliments affecting the toes, skin and sensory organs

Aches Replaces the aching need for recognition through the touch of acceptance.

Acne Releases unexpressed frustration and anger caused by a perceived insecurity at facing the world and replaces them with confidence.

Addictions Provides inner understanding, eliminating the need to escape perceived criticism.

Adenoids Overcomes feelings of inadequacy with recognition of the self.

Aging Eases mind and body so that concern, apprehension and dread no longer wither and shrink the soul.

Alzheimer's disease Provides reassurance that it is safe to exist in the real world without threat to the real self by dismissing the need to escape in the mind.

Amnesia Removes the need to cut off thoughts that threaten personal acceptance or avoid the present and/or past situation.

Anxiety Replaces continual fear with belief and faith in the unlimited support of the universe.

Apathy Instils enthusiasm and re-establishes a purpose for living.

Athlete's foot Removes frustration and irritability by restoring faith in personal concepts and ideas.

Bad breath (Halitosis) Improves inner communication and understanding by clearing foul, festering, revengeful, bitter and wounded thoughts.

Balance (loss of) Centres the mind.

Baldness Releases the intellect from the strain of doubt and uncertainty and eliminates the gripping need for extreme control.

Bell's Palsy Encourages open expression of personal concepts.

Bleeding gums Restores faith and support in personal decisions.

Blindness Replaces the blinding fear of seeing life's circumstances through clear insight.

Brain tumour Dissipates the build-up of accumulated, unexpressed, frustrated and angry thoughts.

Bruising Calms inner turmoil through self-acceptance.

Cancer Removes obstacles to self-development through inner comprehension of contained, upsetting thoughts and emotions.

Cataracts Clears the vision by providing a brighter outlook on life's prospects.

Cerebral palsy Stimulates the thinking process for the lively exchange of ideas.

Cold sores Creates inner peace by eliminating the perceived need to reveal festering, inflamed thoughts.

Coma Replaces the gripping fear of uncertain thoughts with the loving acceptance of life.

Conjunctivitis Soothes the anger and pain of all that is being seen.

Deafness Alerts the inner voice to provide guidance and eliminates the fear of what may be heard.

Depression Provides direction in life and removes the feeling of being in the dark.

Dizziness (Vertigo) Eliminates confusion through clarity of thought.

Dry eyes Encourages the shedding of tears by understanding the difficulty in seeing other points of view.

Earache Eases the pain and hurt at all that is heard, consciously or subconsciously, and replaces it with inner harmony and balance.

Epilepsy Focuses and calms the mind for inner control despite the perceived injustices of life.

Eye disorders Improves insight and clarity of vision revealing the beauty of life.

Fainting Restores faith in personal ability to cope and be in control.

Gum disorders Strengthens belief and support in personal decisions.

Headaches Eases the pain of everything coming to a head and replaces it with feelings of adequacy and a belief in the ability to cope.

Insomnia Soothes the mind so that body and soul can rest easily.

Jaw disorders Reinstates faith and security in personal concepts.

Migraine headaches   Releases the mind from the intense pressure to perform.

Mouth disorders   Encourages open, honest communication within the self regarding personal thoughts and communication with others.

Nervousness   Restores faith and belief in personal capabilities.

Neuralgia   Removes pain and anguish over the rejection of or difficulty in communicating individual ideas.

Nose disorders   Prevents the nose from being knocked out of joint through personal recognition of unique talents and the ability to put them into practice.

Paralysis   Frees the mind from the gripping fear of moving ahead.

Parkinson's disease   Dispels the intense desire to organise others by re-establishing personal control.

Pituitary gland disorders   Restores emotional control and inner harmony.

Seizures   Dissipates profound thoughts from interfering with natural life processes.

Sinus congestion   Relieves accumulated irritability and the perceived need for perfection.

Stroke   Reduces the amount of self-inflicted pressure to meet unrealistically high expectations, making it possible to get ahead with personal concepts and ideas.

Stuttering   Boosts confidence in communicating personal concepts.

Toothache   Removes pain over the making of decisions.

Tinnitus   Alerts the mind to the messages of the inner voice.

Summary

Massage of individual toes stimulates the following thoughts:

Big toes – Personal intellect, intuition and concept.
Second toes – Self-confidence, self-worth and self-esteem.
Third toes – Ideas regarding the pursuit of activities.
Fourth toes – Communication and personal relationships.
Little toes – Expansion and liberation of the mind.

❢ We are what we think. ❡

8

THE TOE NECKS

The neck and throat reflexes in the toe necks reveal the two-way exchange of energies between internal and external environments for open communication so that healthy relationships can form and develop.

Along the bony inner edges of both big toes, between the joints and bases, are the cervical vertebrae reflexes. These mirror the amount of flexibility to pivot the head and see every point of view.

Position of the reflexes on the toe necks

The toe necks, on the soles of the feet, reflect the throat:

- the right toe neck mirrors the right side of the throat revealing past expressions
- the left side of the throat on the left toe neck displays the present exchange of life's expressions.

Bony surfaces on top of the necks reflect the back of the neck revealing the backing and support for honest, open expression of personal concepts and ideas. The degree of flexibility indicates the extent of security in freely expressing and considering all concepts, whilst rigidity due to extreme anxiety and uncertainty restricts mobility leading to single-mindedness.

Impact of tension on the toe neck reflexes

Fear of expressing one's true self tenses the throat and neck muscles, effectively choking and throttling personal individuality. Dread of speaking up arises from:

- apprehension of ridicule
- terror of the consequences
- concern about outside opinion
- trepidation of upsetting others.

When personal creativity is strangled and stifled by social restrictions and expectations, it can lead to anger, guilt or stubbornness, causing:

- lumps of unleashed emotion
- a post-nasal drip from tears that are swallowed for fear of crying openly
- sore throats from the pain and strain of trying to disclose true feelings or from having to swallow or emit angry words.

Insecure thoughts and feelings tense neck muscles and reduce agility. The intense desire to be in control or get ahead may result in:

- a pain in the neck when others threaten personal concepts
- spasm from an extreme urge to be in charge
- stabbing pains from 'getting it in the neck'.

Influence of reflexology on the toe necks

Reflexology massage reflectively:

- soothes and relaxes neck and throat muscles
- creates space for the free flow and exchange of energies
- opens the avenues of expression
- eases internal and external communication.

6 Something we withhold makes us afraid and weak, until we realise that it is ourselves! 9

Reflexology massage of the toe necks

Step 1

- Place both thumbs on the outer edges of the little toe necks with the third fingers directly opposite on top of the little toe necks (Figure 37).
- Gently squeeze the corresponding digits together, and then slowly release until there is only slight contact.
- Lightly rotate the thumbs, whilst resting the third fingers on top (see page 35).

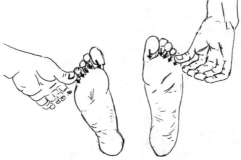

Figure 37 Massage of the toe necks

Step 2

- Move the thumbs fractionally along the little toe necks, still with the third fingers directly opposite, on top.
- Repeat the gentle squeezing, release and rotation technique of Step 1 and continue until all toes necks are completely massaged. Concentrate on the sides of each toe where the greatest tension and emotional congestion are often reflected.

Step 3

- Use the thumbs to gently but firmly stroke the underneath surfaces of all toe necks, from top to bottom, in a milking movement (page 36), starting on the little toes necks and finishing on the big toe necks (Figure 38).

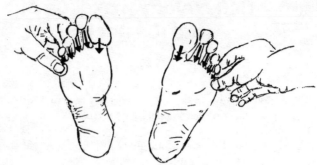

Figure 38 Milking the underneath surface of the toe necks

Step 4

- Repeat Step 3, either with the third fingers or the thumbs on the upper toe neck surfaces (Figure 39).
- Milk the sides and tops of the toe necks particularly well to: ease throat congestion; relieve neck stiffness; reduce cerebral tension.

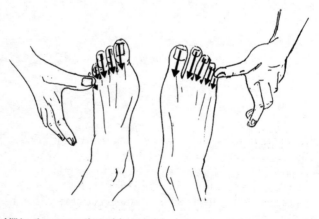

Figure 39 Milking the upper surface of the toe necks

Step 5

- Feather stroke (page 37) the necks of each toe starting on the little toe necks and finishing on the big toe necks, first underneath and then along the tops.

Step 6

- Place all fingers on the tips of the toes and lightly 'walk' them over the tops of the feet to the ankles (Figure 40). Repeat as necessary.

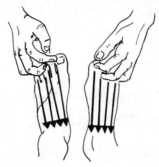

Figure 40 Walking the fingers over the tops of the feet

Stroke both feet from the toes to the ankles a few times and then continue with the massage of the balls of the feet which follows on page 85.

❛ By breaking the mould of social expectation, we discover our own unique identity. ❜

Natural characteristics of the toe necks

Neck and throat reflexes should be firm but flexible with smooth, flesh-coloured skin.

Altered states of the toe neck reflexes

- The effort of trying to express one's true self is reflected through:
  - lines and wrinkles from strain, concern and worry.
  - distinct lines across the throat reflexes from feeling throttled.
  - lumps in the toe necks when feeling choked with emotion.
  - swellings on the sides of the toe necks from post-nasal drip, the swallowed tears of suppressed emotions.

- Skin colouring (see page 45) provides further clues as to the sentiment behind the expression of life, either those things having to be swallowed or openly divulged, or kept retained.

    Red – frustrated, angry or embarrassed.
    White – exhausted.
    Blue to *black* – the degree of hurt.
    Yellow – fed up.
    Green – envious.

Neck and throat disorders eased through reflexology

For all disorders a complete reflexology massage is required concentrating on:

- nervous system and solar plexus reflexes to calm the mind and relieve pain, anxiety and fear.
- endocrine gland reflexes to soothe the emotions and create inner harmony.
- affected gland or organ reflexes to relax the distressed area and ease the symptoms of dis-ease.

Goitre   Reduces the need to project outwards for attention through recognition of one's own individuality.

Hyperthyroidism   Provides space for self-expression.

Hypothyroidism   Boosts self-confidence and re-energises the whole for unique requirements.

Laryngitis   Calms inflamed, angry and frustrated thoughts that have been swallowed and fester in the throat.

Lump in the throat   Reinstates faith in openly expressing true emotions by realising that personal growth and development comes through dealing with perceivably traumatic situations.

Neck problems   Allows flexibility to see every point of view.

Post-nasal drip   Encourages the free flow of tears of joy, pride or grief instead of allowing them to clog the channels of expression.

Sore throat   Provides the courage to speak up for oneself and removes the hurt of others not listening.

Stiff neck   Eliminates the need to put on 'the blinkers' by providing flexibility to see things from every point of view.

Tonsillitis   Boosts belief in personal creativity and encourages the free flow of individuality.

9

THE BALLS OF
THE FEET

The balls of the feet reflect the chest and breast reflexes. They reveal feelings of self-esteem and self-worth that determine the way individuals relate and respond to the constantly changing environment. At birth the first breath indicates initial freedom and independence with the baby's presence demanding space to be an individual in its own right.

Fresh supplies of vital life-forces are absorbed from the external surrounding atmosphere to assist with the internal release of energy for the benefit of mind, body and soul.

Once the advantageous aspects of inhaled air have been utilised, the by-product carbon dioxide is immediately eliminated since it is a potential threat to personal well-being. Carbon dioxide symbolises emotions that have been worked through and are no longer of value to the body.

Within a harmonious, happy environment lungs have an incredible capacity to expand and contract rhythmically to maintain a healthy balance between the acceptance of the beneficial aspects of life and the rejection of threatening substances.

Feelings have an immediate impact on the process, since the exchange of life-forces is directly related to the nurturing process via the breasts. Enhanced feelings expand the chest, whilst crushing emotions are deflating.

Position of the reflexes on the — balls of the feet and the effect of — reflexology on these reflexes

Beneath the necks of the toes on the balls of both feet are the shoulder reflexes (Figure 41). Through reflexology these are strengthened to carry the responsibility of enjoying life to the full.

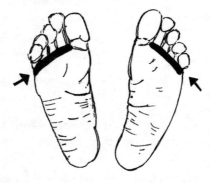

Figure 41 The shoulder reflexes

On the lower inner crease of both big toe necks are the thyroid gland reflexes (Figure 42). As their butterfly shape implies, space is required to spread the wings for expression of one's true self, encouraged through massage.

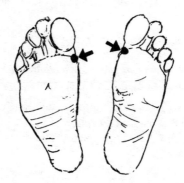

Figure 42 The thyroid gland reflexes

Beneath the thyroid reflexes about halfway down the balls of both feet are the thymus gland reflexes (Figure 43). These are slightly swollen mounds in the very young and elderly, but are hollow in adults.

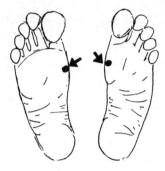

Figure 43 The thymus gland reflexes

As the seat of the soul, the thymus gland protects and shields the body from outside attack by producing killer cells that destroy any threatening forces.

Reflexology strengthens the immune system by inflating feelings of self-worth and self-esteem that are impenetrable to outside attack. Spend time on these reflexes during periods of vulnerability and emotional distress, such as a broken relationship, death or retrenchment.

The oesophagus reflexes extend from the mouth reflexes, on the inner joints of the big toes, along the inner edges of the toe necks and balls of both feet, to the base of the hard skin of the balls (Figure 44). Reflexology massage facilitates the ability to swallow life's experiences with ease.

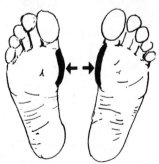

Figure 44 Oesophagus reflexes

The upper arm and knee reflexes on the outer edges of the balls of both feet enjoy the freedom provided by reflexology to expand and fully embrace the enormity of life (Figure 45).

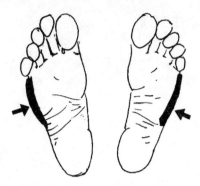

Figure 45 Upper arm and knee reflexes

The bulk of the balls of the feet contain the lung reflexes (Figure 46) which, when massaged:

- create space for feelings of well-being and self-enhancement
- encourage effortless adaption to constantly changing atmospheric conditions
- give and take with ease.

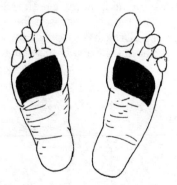

Figure 46 Lung reflexes

The breast reflexes (Figure 47) overlap the lung reflexes to provide nourishment for self-development. The size of breasts indicate the amount of nourishment given and received:

- large bosoms have a tremendous capacity to nurture but reach out for more affection to boost personal feelings of self-worth and value
- flattened mammary glands are drained and exhausted from either caring so much for others to the detriment of oneself, or withholding the nurturing process due to withdrawal from a perceived lack of self-esteem.

Reflexology provides adequate sustenance for all concerned and inflates personal feelings of unconditional love.

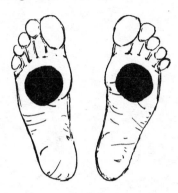

Figure 47 Breast reflexes

Below the balls of both feet in the centres are the solar plexus reflexes (Figure 48). These emotional centres are also known as the 'abdominal brain' since feelings have immediate impact on the digestive process.

The solar plexus reflexes are the most powerful reflexes on the feet. Body, mind and soul can be immediately calmed through them. Incredible serenity and peace created throughout can effectively:

- ease anxiety and panic attacks
- relieve an asthmatic bronchial spasm
- calm palpitations
- reduce hysteria
- regulate hyperventilation.

At the base of the balls of both feet, on the inner edges, are the heart reflexes (Figure 49), the bulk of which are on the left foot. Reflexology strengthens and purifies affections, opening the heart to unconditional love of oneself and others.

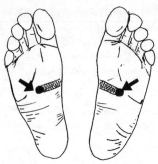

Figure 48 Solar plexus reflexes

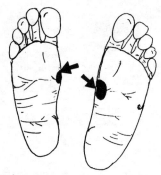

Figure 49 Heart reflexes

On top of the feet, over the balls of both feet, are the reflexes for back of the ribcage. These reinforce and back emotions effectively when stimulated through reflexology.

The impact of tension on the balls of the feet reflexes

Feelings, emotions and exercise immediately alter the breathing mechanism:

- excitement and exercise speed up the rate
- disturbing emotions such as fear and anxiety suppress the breath
- when upset, long deep breaths are taken in and short sobs emitted
- life-threatening situations temporarily halt breathing.

The influence of reflexology on the balls of the feet

Reflexology massage on the balls of the feet liberates the breath by relaxing the ribcage so that the lungs can expand freely to accommodate the fullness of life. Excessive tension and entrapped heavy emotions are released, taking a weight off the chest. The sense of relief can be overwhelming.

Through reflexology massage latent contents of emotional congestion can be subconsciously unravelled and released to eliminate feelings of frustration, bewilderment and fear.

❝ Within our reach lies every path we ever dream of taking,
Within our power lies every step that we ever dream of making,
Within our range lies every joy we ever dream of seeing,
Within ourselves lies everything we ever dream of being. ❞

Reflexology massage of the balls of the feet

Step 1

● Place the thumbs on the outer edges of the balls of the feet, immediately below both little toes, with the third fingers situated directly above, on top of the feet (Figure 50).

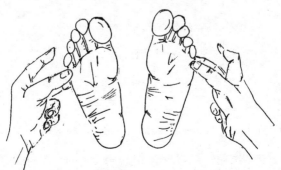

Figure 50 Position of the thumbs and fingers on the balls of the feet

Step 2

- Gently squeeze the corresponding thumbs and third fingers together, apply slight pressure and then release.
- Without moving position, lightly rotate the thumbs on the spot, with the third fingers resting gently on top (see rotation technique page 35).

Step 3

- Move both thumbs fractionally along the horizontal strips, staying beneath the necks of the little toes, with the third fingers following directly above.
- Repeat Step 2 and then move the digits fractionally along and continue to massage the strips along the tops of the balls of the feet, at the base of the toe necks, until you reach the big toes.
- Massage these strips several times, especially if hard or swollen, to ease the load of perceived burdens and responsibilities that are being shouldered.

Step 4

- Milk the strips by placing the digits immediately below the little toe necks and sliding them firmly but gently along the bases of both little toe necks into the gaps between the little and fourth toes (Figure 51). Then slide the digits beneath the fourth toe necks into the gaps between the fourth and third toes.

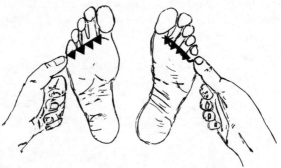

Figure 51 Scalloping movement on the shoulder reflexes

- Continue this scalloping movement beneath each toe neck until you reach the gaps between the second and big toes. Repeat Step 4 from the beginning, if necessary.

Step 5

- Position the thumbs and third fingers fractionally below the starting point of Step 1 and repeat the movements in Step 2 (Figure 52).
- After massaging each horizontal strip, lower the position of the digits, on the outer edges of the balls of both feet, and continue the massage until the balls of both feet have been thoroughly stimulated.

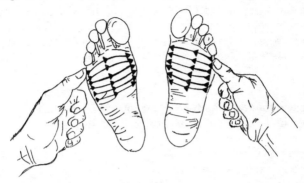

Figure 52 Massaging the balls of the feet

Step 6

- Return to Steps 1 and 2 but this time massage in vertical strips from below the little toe necks to the bases of the balls of the feet, from top to bottom (Figure 53).
- Repeat under the fourth toes, then in strips beneath the third toes, followed by the second toes, and finally the big toes until both balls are thoroughly massaged.

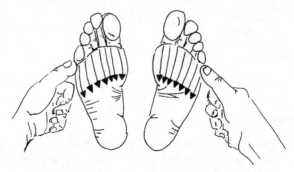

Figure 53 Massaging the vertical strips on the balls of the feet

Step 7

- Repeat Step 6, but this time slide the digits down the balls of the feet from beneath the necks of the little toes, along the outer edge, to the base   of the balls of both feet in a milking movement (page 35).

Step 8

- Feather stroke (page 37) the balls of the feet with an exceptionally light touch, using either the fronts or the backs of the second fingers. Begin beneath the little toes and feather stroke in vertical strips, from top to bottom, from the outer edges to the inner borders of both feet.

Step 9

- Repeat the feather stroke on the tops, opposite the balls of both feet. Reflexology massage of the balls of the feet:
  - provides space to breathe
  - gets emotions off the chest
  - boosts feelings of self-worth
  - encourages the nurturing process.

Step 10

- To massage the upper arm reflexes place the thumbs or preferred digits immediately beneath the little toes and use the caterpillar or rotation movements (page 35), starting on the bony swellings, continuing along the bony ridges on the perimeters of both feet to end at the bony protrusions half way down the feet (Figure 54).

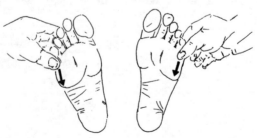

Figure 54 Upper arm reflexes

(The bony swellings reflect the shoulder sockets; the ridge of bone represents the upper arms; the midway bony protrusions mirror the elbow reflexes.)

- Then thoroughly milk all reflexes and finally feather stroke the areas to release the upper arms from constraining circumstances that pin them down.

Step 11

- To locate the knee reflexes, place the thumbs on the shoulder reflexes and the third fingers on the elbow reflexes and allow the second fingers to touch the mid-points between the two, at a slightly higher level (Figure 55). (The bony ledge reflects the flattened surface of a bent knee; the knee is also reflected onto the central points of the balls of both feet, over the nipple reflexes.)
- Reflexology encourages the knees to be flexible and change direction with ease.

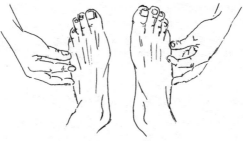

Figure 55 Locating the knee reflexes

Step 12

- Place the thumbs on the lower creases beneath the big toes, with the third fingers placed directly above on top of the feet (Figure 56). These are the thyroid gland reflexes and are stimulated to create space for personal expression.

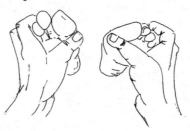

Figure 56 Massaging thyroid gland reflexes

- Gently squeeze thumbs and third fingers together and hold for a few seconds. Slightly release the pressure, then lightly rotate the thumbs without moving the position of the digits. Continue to ease the compression until barely touching the skin's surface. Rest the digits in this position for a few seconds.
- Remove both thumbs and lightly rest the third fingers on the thyroid reflexes for a few seconds. This encourages gushes of energy to revitalise and balance the glands.
- Visualisation of the colour turquoise blue enhances the effect.
- Gently stroke both reflexes.

Step 13

- Place the thumbs about halfway down the inner edges of the balls of the feet, with the third fingers directly opposite on the tops of the feet (Figure 57).
- Feel for slight hollows in adults and possible swellings in babies, youngsters and the elderly. These are the thymus gland reflexes and are stimulated for increased self-esteem and self-confidence.

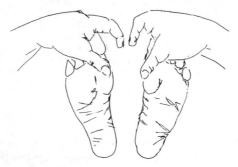

Figure 57 Massaging thymus gland reflexes

- Gently squeeze thumbs and third fingers together and hold for a few seconds. Slightly release the pressure and lightly rotate the thumbs without moving position. Continue to ease off and then, with the skin surfaces barely touching, rest the digits without movement for a few seconds.
- Remove the thumbs and replace with the tips of the third fingers. Rest the third fingers on the thymus reflexes to balance and re-energise the gland.

- Visualisation of the colour green enhances the effect. Finish by lightly stroking the reflexes.

Step 14

- Now, very lightly place the tips of the second or third fingers on the heart reflexes, on the inner surfaces of both feet, at the bases of the balls of the feet (Figure 58).
- Gently rotate the tips, visualising green, and then rest the digits without movement for a few seconds.
- Lovingly stroke these sensitive reflexes.

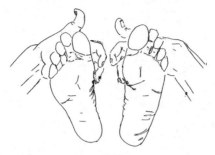

Figure 58 Massaging the heart reflexes

Step 15

- Massage the inner edges in strips from beneath the necks of the big toes to the bases of the balls of the feet, first with several caterpillar or rotation movements, then a few milking movements and finally feather stroke the areas thoroughly (Figure 59). The oesophagus and airway reflexes accept and exchange vital life-forces more easily when relaxed.

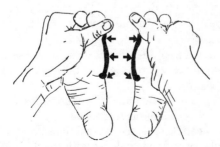

Figure 59 Massaging oesophagus and airway reflexes

Step 16

- Again place the thumbs or fingers immediately below the necks of the big toes but this time on the ridge of bone.
- Massage with the caterpillar or rotation movements several times from the big toe necks to the base of the balls of both feet, then milk and finally feather stroke to boost emotional support for inner strength (Figure 60).

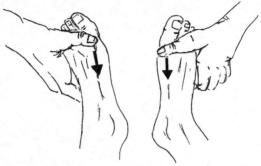

Figure 60 Massaging the upper back reflexes

Step 17

Massaging the solar plexus reflexes

These are the most important reflexes on the feet and can be used, particularly in an emergency, to immediately calm an agitated, fearful state.

- Place the thumbs on the central indentations immediately below the balls of both feet, with the third fingers resting on the opposite reflexes on top of the feet to intensify the effect (Figure 61). Remove the third fingers if the energies feel too overpowering.
- Without movement apply gentle but firm pressure with the thumbs only until a slight resistance is felt. At this point allow all digits to rest for a few seconds.
- Slowly ease the compression until the thumbs barely touch the skin's surface. Stay still for as long as necessary.
- This movement can be repeated several times, if required.
- Stroke the reflexes and then balance with the third fingers directly on the two points on both soles.

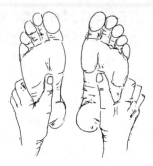

Figure 61 Massaging the solar plexus reflexes

Step 18

● Massage the tops, over the balls of both feet to strengthen the back of the ribcage for greater emotional backing.

Step 19

● The bony ridges along the inside edges of the balls of both feet, above the fleshy instep reflect the upper thoracic vertebrae and upper spine reflexes which are strengthened through massage to give greater emotional support.

Stroke both feet from toes to ankles and then massage the instep reflexes (page 106).

> ❛ If we wish for kindness,
> We need to be kind to ourselves,
> If we yearn for the truth
> We need to be true to ourselves,
> For what we give of ourselves,
> Is always reflected back. ❜

Natural characteristics of the balls of the feet

The balls of the feet are naturally flesh-coloured mounds that occupy the upper third of the soles immediately below the toe necks. Their flexibility and colour allow them to adapt and blend into any environment and ever-changing atmosphere with ease.

Altered states of the balls of the feet reflexes

- The constant variation of colours on the balls of the feet reveal fluctuating emotions that continually surface as thoughts evoke feelings:

  Red –   embarrassed, frustrated or angry.
  White –   drained of energy, tired and exhausted.
  Black / blue –   the various shades display the depth of emotional hurt and bruised feelings.
  Yellow / orange – feeling fed up.

The position of the colouring on the balls of the feet is significant, depending on the reflex.

- Swellings immediately below the toe necks, along the shoulder reflexes, reveal the perceived weight of burdens and responsibility carried on the shoulders. Faith in universal support eases the load.
- Thyroid gland reflexes on the lower inner crease of the necks of both big toes:
  - **distend** when reaching for more time and space and time for sole and soul expression
  - **diminish** through exhaustion from doing so much for others
  - **harden** to resist or conceal true personal expression
  - **develop** hard skin to protect individuality.
- Oesophagus reflexes, which extend along the inner edges from the mouth reflexes on the pads of the big toes to the base of the balls, develop a ridge of hard skin:
  - when life is hard to swallow, or
  - to conceal true feelings regarding life's circumstances.
- Upper arm reflexes on the outer edges of the balls of both feet:
  - Swell when trying to break free from:
    - inhibiting or overwhelming emotions, especially within the family, or
    - an emotionally fraught environment.
  - Develop hard skin over the swellings to conceal this desire.
- Lung and the overlapping breast reflexes on the balls of the feet:
  - enlarge when weighed down with emotions kept close to the chest or when reaching out for love and affection

– flatten from feeling winded, deflated or drained of self- nourishment, self-esteem and loving feelings
– wrinkle with concern about feelings and atmospheric conditions
– are marked and lined from emotional impact on personal regard
– harden or develop callouses to protect, shield or conceal perceived detrimental feelings that may drain or threaten self-worth
– form bunions in an attempt to break the bounds of rigid belief systems that stifle emotions and entrap the soul, robbing it of its individuality.
- Thymus gland reflexes, immediately below the thyroid gland reflexes, roughly halfway down the balls of the feet:
    – bulge to provide extra protection when feeling vulnerable, or when reaching out for personal recognition
    – subside from the exhaustion of having to defend oneself from emotional abuse and perceived criticism
    – develop hard skin to form a shield against perceived attack at soul level.
- Solar plexus reflexes at the base of the balls of both feet:
    – inflate when overcome with heavy feelings
    – deflate from being drained of emotion
    – carry the lines and marks of inner turmoil and division.
- Heart reflexes, on the inner edges of both feet, at the base of the balls of the feet:
    – enlarge when filled with heartfelt issues or when reaching out for unconditional love and affection
    – fade when drained or disillusioned with the process of love
    – develop tiny blood blisters when the heart is broken
    – form hard skin to protect against being stabbed in the heart.
- Back of the ribcage reflexes on the tops of the feet opposite the balls become:
    – taut with strained ligaments when:
        – feeling under emotional pressure
        – seeking extra strength
        – trying to support or prop up oneself within the environment
    – puffy with unshed tears.
- Upper thoracic vertebrae, upper spine reflexes, on the bony ridges along the inside edges of the balls of both feet:
    – collapse through a perceived lack of emotional support
    – bulge to display a need for extra strength and emotional backing.

Respiratory and circulatory disorders

Respiratory and circulatory disorders occur when:

- vibrancy for life is diminished through lack of enthusiasm
- feeling emotionally disillusioned
- heartfelt feelings are kept close to the chest
- deflated and exhausted from nurturing others
- lacking self-esteem and self-worth
- unconditional love for the self and others is diminished
- greed and insensitivity are prominent
- true sentiments are concealed behind a smoke screen
- feeling vulnerable and attacked
- suffocated by overwhelming situations
- unable to breathe for the self
- creativity and individuality are suppressed.

Specific respiratory and circulatory ailments eased through reflexology

For any disorder a complete reflexology massage is required with greater attention to:

- nervous system and solar plexus reflexes to calm the mind and relieve pain, anxiety and fear
- endocrine gland reflexes to soothe the emotions and create inner harmony
- affected gland or organ reflexes to relax the distressed area and ease the symptoms of dis-ease.

The following also includes disorders affecting the chest, upper back and limbs.

Aids Replaces feelings of inadequacy with belief in self-worth and value within society.

Allergies Calms extreme sensitivity, irritability and vulnerability by increasing the level of tolerance.s

Anaemia   Replenishes inner strength by boosting self-worth.

Arteries   Fills the blood vessels with renewed enthusiasm to nurture all cells for personal growth and development.

Arteriosclerosis   Releases the arteries from perceived pressures, hardness and distrust of life.

Asphyxiating attacks   Removes the panic of being overwhelmed and suffocated and replaces it with faith in the expansiveness of life.

Asthma   Makes space for the individual to breathe without feeling smothered by an over-concerned or overpowering parent. Otherwise overcome with breathtaking emotion.

Bleeding   Replaces sadness with love and joy.

Blood pressure   Maintains a harmonious flow of love and joy throughout. High blood pressure: dissolves accumulated tension from unresolved emotional issues. Low blood pressure: boosts the flow of love and joy through self-acceptance.

Blood clotting   Opens the channels of communication.

Blood disorders   Creates inner harmony for the unimpeded flow of happiness.

Breast cysts   Dispenses with contained emotions of anger and the frustration at either not receiving enough or giving too much nourishment.

Breathing disorders   Dispels feelings of inadequacy and expands self-esteem.

Bronchitis   Eliminates frustration and anger at the threat to personal well-being within the environment.

Bunions   Liberates entrapped, contained emotions.

Carpel tunnel syndrome   Relieves distress by making life easier to handle and manage.

Cholesterol   Reinstates faith in the loving process by removing the gripping fear or distrust of emotional commitment.

Circulation   Inner peace and unconditional acceptance of oneself enhance the flow and distribution of life-forces for overall nurturing.

Colds   Unleashes repressed rage by letting go of past irritations. The end of a cold marks the beginning of a new cycle.

Congestion   Circulation is re-established removing all obstacles so that the natural flow of life-forces is enhanced throughout.

Emphysema   Boosts self-esteem and self-worth by providing the courage to live to the full.

Heartburn   Releases the gripping fear of heartfelt issues.

Hyperventilation   Calms inner panic.

Increased blood acidity Replaces fear, worry and anxiety with faith and unconditional love for oneself and others.

Increased white blood cells Naturally fortifies the body, mind and soul during periods of perceived personal abuse and attack.

Knee disorders Inflates feelings about oneself so that changes in direction are facilitated and progress made.

Leukaemia Releases unexpressed anger and frustration at the lack of unconditional love and joy, due to unrealistic pressures.

Lung disorders Fills the whole with appreciation of oneself creating contentment within the environment.

Mastitis Calms anger and frustration at the emotional demands of others or at perceived lack of being appreciated.

Pneumonia Heals emotional hurts and fills the whole with enthusiasm for life.

Round shoulders Lifts perceived burdens of responsibility from the shoulders for appropriate emotional responses.

Sickle cell anaemia Makes room for unconditional love by removing restrictions that inhibit the full expression of joy.

Thymus disorders Reinforces inner strength by reducing vulnerability with the belief that nothing and no one is a threat unless allowed to be.

Upper back problems Strengthens emotional backing and support through unconditional love and acceptance of oneself.

Varicose veins Replaces the weight and burdens of disagreeable situations and hopeless discouragement with an enthusiasm for the direction and circumstances of life.

10
THE INSTEPS

The insteps reflect the bulk of the digestive tract and its related organs, as well as part of the excretory and reproductive systems.

Position of the reflexes on the insteps and the effect of reflexology on these reflexes

The triangular mound that occupies the upper outer quadrant of the right fleshy instep is the bulk of the liver reflex (Figure 62). The tip extends slightly onto the left foot to overlap a portion of the stomach reflexes.

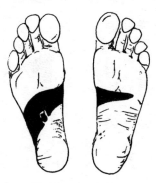

Figure 62 Liver and gall bladder reflexes

Reflexology keeps the liver in a harmonious state of well-being so that, being the largest and most versatile organ in the body, it can perform its numerous functions effectively and efficiently. It is able to:

- store abundant energy
- actively provide fuel for the physical expression and manifestation of ideas and feelings
- generate sufficient bodily heat for ideal warmth
- detoxify threatening elements
- modify chemical substances
- act as a reservoir for blood.
- The gall bladder reflex (Figure 62) is a tiny round swelling towards the centre of the instep on the right foot. Massage of this reflex encourages the bile to pass into the duodenum and assist with the beneficial breakdown of fats. This prevents the accumulation of bitterness.
- Pancreas gland reflexes (Figure 63) are situated just above the 'waistline' of both feet, extending from the centres of the inner edges of both insteps. Reflexology assists the pancreas in maintaining a favourable sugary environment to provide energy and enthusiasm for all activities.
- The reflex of the spleen (Figure 63), on the outer upper left instep, is massaged to determine that all actions are accomplished with the appropriate amount of precision.

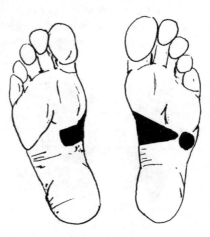

Figure 63 Pancreas and splenic reflexes

- The stomach reflexes occupy the bulk of the upper inner quadrant of the left instep with part of the reflex being on the corresponding area on the right instep (Figure 64). Reflexology makes it easier to stomach life's experiences through the effective breakdown and transformation of food into acceptable nutritional components.

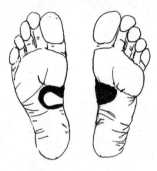

Figure 64 The stomach and duodenum reflexes

- The 'C' shaped reflex on the upper inner quadrant of the right instep is the duodenal reflex (Figure 64) Massage of this reflex encourages the effortless movement of food from the stomach to theintestines. Nutritional substances are converted further in the duodenum by bile from the gall bladder and pancreatic juices from the pancreas.
- The adrenal reflexes are immediately below the solar plexus reflexes, with the right adrenal reflex being slightly lower and more central than the left adrenal reflex (Figure 65). Reflexology massage of the adrenal reflexes ensures super-human strength during life-threatening situations.

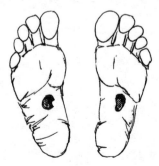

Figure 65 The adrenal and kidney reflexes

- Kidney reflexes (Figure 65 are tiny vertical mounds beneath the adrenal reflexes. Massage of these reflexes encourages the kidney to filter and ourify the blood contents effciently and effectively to ensure a harmonious chemical environment and the correct fluid balance.
- Small intestine (Figure 66) reflexes occupy the lower halves of both insteps. Massage of these assists in the absorption of beneficial nutrients to energise the whole for personal growth and the development of new bodily cells.

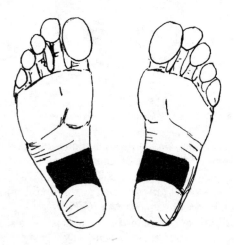

Figure 66 Small intestine reflexes

- The large intestine or colon reflexes (Figure 67) contain remnants of the past and waste substances. It is reflected along the borders of the lower halves of the insteps.
  - The ascending colon is reflected vertically along the lower half of the outer border of the right foot only, between the fleshy instep and the harder thicker edge.
  - The transverse colon reflexes are contained within the horizontal strip that crosses the centre of both insteps.
  - The descending colon is reflected vertically along the lower half of the outer border, on the left foot only, between the fleshy instep and the harder outer edge.
  - The sigmoid colon reflex, only on the left foot, follows the bound ary between the left instep and left heel.

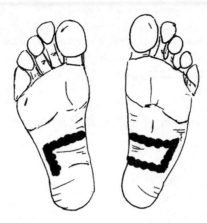

Figure 67 Colon reflexes

● The reflexes of the female reproductive organs and glands (Figure 68):
  – uterus reflexes are on the lower inside edges of the instep
  – fallopian tubes and fingers reflexes stretch across the bases of
    both insteps
  – the ovaries reflexes are in the outer lower corners of the insteps.

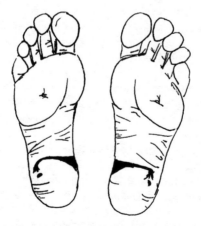

Figure 68 Reflexes of the female reproductive organs and glands

Massage encourages acceptance of the female role to create, accommodate and nurture new life.

- The ridge of the bone along the inner edges of both feet reflect the lumbar vertebrae, the middle spine (see Figure 88). Massage of these reflexes boosts support for all activities and communication.
- Centre back reflexes directly above the fleshy instep on the tops of the feet, have their backing for all activities and relationships reinforced through reflexology.

Impact of tension on the instep reflexes

The digestive process is heavily influenced by all types of emotion from extreme ecstasy to anger, fear, excitement, nervousness, insecurity and so on. The digestive tract reacts in the following ways to tension:

- the harmonious expansion and contraction of the alimentary canal is upset
- the progress of food is hampered
- strained, adverse conditions cause irritability.

Excessive fat acts as a shock absorber against perceived emotional attack or as a cover-up of the true self.

- The liver becomes frustrated and angry when continually pressurised into doing things to please others:
  - a distended liver reflex stores turbulent emotions
  - a sunken liver reflex is exhausted from being pressurised into meeting social and family expectations.
- The gall bladder reflex hardens with accumulated bitterness at having to carry out particular actions. For example, an increase of gall stones during war years reveal built-up resentment at having to act under orders.
- Pancreatic reflexes bulge to reach out to find joy and enthusiasm for life's activities. Deflated reflexes display exhaustion at continually doing things to please others. Pancreatic disorders generally occur soon after a traumatic event that robs the individual of the pleasures in life.
- The reflex of the spleen enlarges with obsessive behaviour or when there is specific need to prove something to family or society. It sinks when unable to stand up to strict rules and unrealistic expectations.

- The stomach is upset by:
  - deep dread
  - extreme concern
  - fear of new circumstances
  - inability to cope.
- Adrenal reflexes inflate when extremely fearful or anxious about a perceived life-threatening situation, and flatten when feeling defeated.
- Hardened kidney reflexes reflect perceived disappointments and swell when overwhelmed by the enormity of it all, or deflate when drained of enthusiasm.
- Excessive fear and lack of self-worth flatten the small intestine reflexes, depriving them of their vibrancy, whereas concern and worry cause them to wrinkle.
- The reflexes of the large intestine or colon dread failure and long for recognition of personal abilities.
  - Transverse colon reflexes swell when competing against oneself or when placed under pressure to perform better than personal best.
- The reflexes of the female uterus:
  - look bruised or have many small broken blood vessels when there is perceived abuse of femineity, either physical or emotional
  - swell and turn red when disappointed and frustrated at not falling pregnant
  - appear battered if unable to get ahead in a male-dominated society.
- Prominent bony swellings over the central spine reflexes are affectionately referred to as 'guilt bumps':
  - prominent swellings on the upper part of the central vertebrae reflexes reveal perceived shame over actions
  - bony prominences over the lower part of the central vertebral reflexes reflect regret regarding relationships.

  These bumps can disappear with the knowledge that life is a journey of unexpected learning experiences from which wisdom can be acquired.

Influence of reflexology on the insteps

Reflexology calms the digestive process and eliminates edginess, anxiety and fear. As a result, life circumstances become:

- manageable, making it possible to cope with all that is on one's plate
- palatable due to improved taste
- delightful to chew
- easier to swallow
- pleasant to stomach
- agreeable to absorb
- gratifying to let go of wasteful aspects.

With regular massage, hunger becomes the strongest desire to grow, develop and survive.

When relaxed and at ease, appropriate amounts and types of food are naturally chosen to replenish, nourish and refuel mind, body and soul with life-sustaining forces that provide balance in life.

Reflexology assists in taking a weight off the mind and body by releasing heavy emotions weighing down the whole. The perceived need to conceal and cover up the true self with excessive fat diminishes as self-confidence grows to replace uncertainty and fear.

Reflexology provides a healthy appetite for life, as well as the energy and enthusiasm to enjoy it.

Reflexology massage of the instep reflexes

The bulk of the digestive organ reflexes are reflected onto the fleshy insteps, but reflexology massage of the digestive tract begins at the mouth reflexes in the big toes and ends in the anal reflexes on the inner heels.

Step 1

- Place both thumbs or third fingers on the mouth reflexes, on the inner edges of the big toes, just below the joints (Figure 69).
- Apply slight pressure and gently rotate the digits to facilitate the chewing process and to improve the sense of taste.

Step 2

- Using the caterpillar or rotation technique (page 34), massage the vertical strips down the inner surfaces of the balls of both feet to harmonise the peristaltic action and facilitate swallowing through the throat and down the oesophagus (Figure 70).

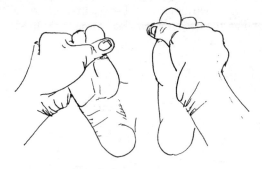

Figure 69 Massaging the mouth reflexes

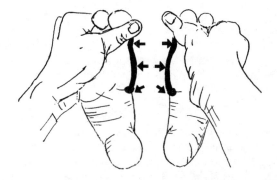

Figure 70 Massaging throat, oesophagus and cardiac sphincter reflexes

Step 3

- Rest the digits on the slight swellings at the junction of the balls of the feet and the insteps, on the reflexes of the cardiac sphincter, at the entrance of the stomach (Figure 71).
- Apply slight pressure, hold for a few seconds and then slowly release.
- Gently massage and finish by stroking lightly.

These reflexes require extra attention for those suffering from heartburn or hiatus hernia.

Step 4

- Visualise the stomach reflex on the left foot and thoroughly massage with the caterpillar or rotation technique (page 34). Use the left digit to massage in horizontal strips from left to right, and use the right digit to massage horizontally from right to left (Figure 71).
- Repeat on the small stomach reflex on the right foot.

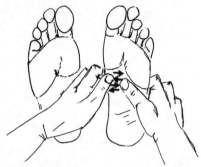

Figure 71 Massaging stomach reflexes

This movement facilitates the breakdown of food and enhances personal belief in the ability to cope with current situations.

Step 5

- Still on the right instep, massage in a C-shaped movement, following the perimeter of the upper inner quadrant (Figure 72).
- Facilitate the procedure by changing digits midway around the C.
- This is the reflex of the duodenum where food is further assimilated.

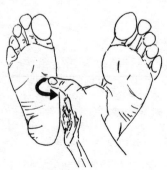

Figure 72 Massaging the duodenum reflex

Step 6

- With the left digit continue across the central line of the left instep, over the ileum reflex to facilitate the passage of nutrients from the duodenum to the small intestine (Figure 73).

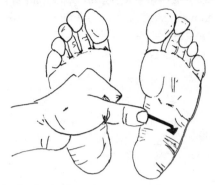

Figure 73 Massaging the Ileum reflex

Step 7

- Now massage in horizontal strips from right to left with the right digit and then left to right with the left digit, across both insteps, until the lower half of both insteps are thoroughly massaged (Figure 74).
- Reflexology ensures the efficient absorption of nutrients in the small intestines.

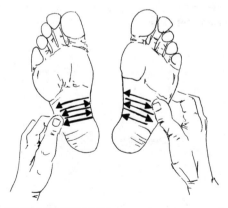

Figure 74 Massaging small intestine reflexes

Step 8

- Complete Step 7 with the right digit in the lower left corner of the right instep and replace with the left digit pointing upwards (Figure 75).
- Massage the lower half of the outer edge of the right instep to facilitate the movement of life's remnants up the ascending colon reflex. Pause halfway up the instep.

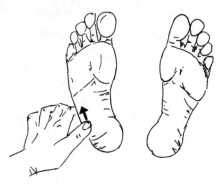

Figure 75 Massaging the ascending colon reflexes

Step 9

- At this midway point, turn the digit so that it is pointing to the right (Figure 76).
- Massage across the centre of both insteps from the left to the right to release the pressure of high expectations that can swell these transverse colon reflexes.

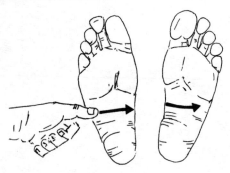

Figure 76 Massaging transverse colon reflexes

Step 10

- At the outer edge of the left instep, replace the left digit with the right one pointing downwards (Figure 77).
- Massage down the border of the outer edge of the instep to the heel to soothe the descending colon for the continued journey of unwanted substances.

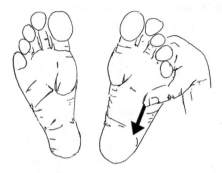

Figure 77 Massaging the descending colon reflex

Step 11

- Now massage from right to left along the lower horizontal strip of the left instep, immediately above the left heel (Figure 78).
- This is the sigmoid colon reflex which may swell when there is an accumulation of wasted emotions that are about to be finally dispensed with.

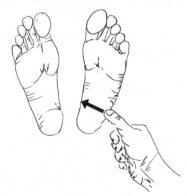

Figure 78 Massaging the sigmoid colon reflex

Step 12

- Place both digits on each foot at the junction of the heel and instep, on the inner edges of both feet (Figure 79).
- Massage in an arc around the mound on the inner edges of both feet to the slight indentations midway between the inner ankles and inside heel tips.
- These are the rectum and anus reflexes which require extra attention for constipation, diarrhoea, haemorrhoids or diverticulitis.

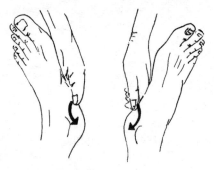

Figure 79 Massaging the rectum reflexes

Step 13

- Rest both digits on the slight indentations, midway between the inner ankles and inside heel tips to boost the energy flow and strengthen the anal sphincters (Figure 80).

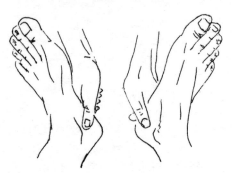

Figure 80 Massaging anal sphincter reflexes

Step 14

- Repeat Steps 1 to 13 using the milking movement (page 35) to soothe emotions and create inner peace for the harmonious expansion and contraction of the alimentary canal.
- Repeat steps 1 to 13, this time massaging with the feather stroke movement (page 36) to re-establish contact with one's true self.

Step 15

- Place the thumbs either side of the insteps, immediately below the balls of both feet, to massage and invigorate the triangular liver reflex on the right foot (Figure 62) and the circular spleen reflex (Figure 63) on the left foot. Milk and then feather stroke.
- Use all three techniques to massage the pancreas reflexes (Figure 63), immediately above the waistline, for a balanced sugary environment.

Step 16

- Place both digits immediately below the solar plexus reflexes, with the left digit situated fractionally further in and very slightly further down than the right digit, on the adrenal gland reflexes (Figure 81).
- Rotate the tips of both digits whilst applying slight pressure on the reflexes.
- Very slowly release the compression and then rest both digits, without movement, on the reflexes.
- Gently place the tips of the third fingers on these points and hold for a few seconds.

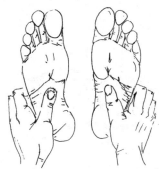

Figure 81 Massaging adrenal gland reflexes

- Reflexology alerts the adrenal glands to respond only to actual rather than imagined life-threatening events so the body is less uptight and highly strung.

Step 17

- Replace the preferred digit on the adrenal reflexes pointing downwards towards the heel (Figure 82).
- Massage the two tiny vertical strips, immediately below, with either the caterpillar or rotation techniques.
- Milk and then feather stroke these kidney reflexes.
- The kidneys filter and eliminate toxic substances from the blood that are detrimental to inner harmony. In this way balance is maintained for purification of the mind, body and soul.

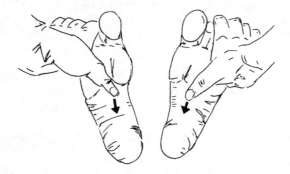

Figure 82 Massaging kidney reflexes

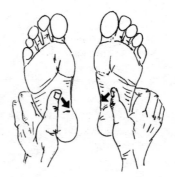

Figure 83 Massaging ureter reflexes

Step 18

- From the mid-point of the kidney reflexes massage in strips along the ureter reflexes to the swollen mounds at the bases of the insteps on the inner edges of both feet (Figure 83).

Step 19

- Now massage the mounds on the inside edges (Figure 84).
- These are the reflexes of the bladder which act as reservoirs of urine and swell considerably when personal relationships cause unhappiness.
- Massage both reflexes thoroughly to facilitate the release of discarded emotions.

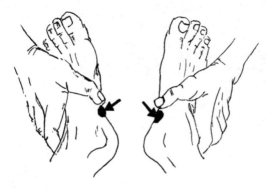

Figure 84 Massaging bladder reflexes

Step 20

- Now massage the urethra reflexes on the inner aspects of both feet:
  - The female urethra reflexes end at the slight indentations midway between the inner ankle and heel tip (Figure 85).
  - The male urethra reflexes extend to the tips of both heels (Figure 86).
- Reflexology strengthens the two muscular sphincters of the urethra, at the base of the bladder and at the outlet, for the effective control of urine. Massage these reflexes particularly well:
  - during periods of insecurity
  - for enuresis (bed wetting)
  - for incontinence.

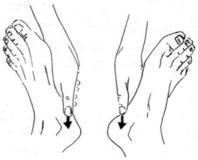

Figure 85 Massaging female urethra reflexes

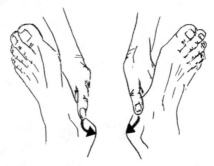

Figure 86 Massaging male urethra reflexes

Step 21

Repeat Steps 17 to 20, first with milking movements to soothe the flow of urine, and then with feather strokes to reaffirm basic security through inner control.

Step 22

- Place the left fingers on the outer edge of the right foot and the right fingers on the outside edge of the left foot, either side of the middle portions of both feet (Figure 87).
- 'Walk' all the fingers in unison over the tops of both feet to massage the reflexes that back both insteps and to strengthen the backing for all activities and relationships.
- Repeat several times and then lightly run the tips of the fingers over the tops of both feet, from the toes to the ankles.

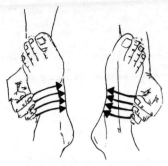

Figure 87 Walking the fingers over the instep

Step 23

● Massage the softer inner edges of the insteps on the insides of both feet, first with strips of the caterpillar or rotation movement, then thoroughly milk, and finally feather stroke.

Step 24

● With caterpillar or rotation movements massage the bony ridges of the spinal reflexes, along the inner edges of both insteps, from the base of the balls of the feet to the start of the heels (Figure 88).
● Repeat several times, then milk and finally, lightly feather stroke both reflexes. This strengthens support and backing for all activities and relationships.

Lightly stroke both feet, top and bottom, from toes to ankles, concentrating on the instep reflexes. Then massage the heels.

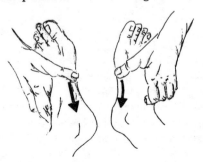

Figure 88 Massaging middle spine reflexes

❛ Think only the best, do only the best, expect only the best. ❜

Natural characteristics of the instep reflexes

The soft insteps are naturally flesh-coloured, vibrant, flexible areas, in the central part of the soles on both feet:

- the upper half of the right instep reflects thoughts and feelings regarding past activities
- the upper portion of the left instep reflects present concepts of personal pursuits
- the lower half of the right instep reveals situations regarding past relationships
- the left lower instep mirrors the state of communications in the present.

Altered states of the instep reflexes

- The colours of the insteps demonstrate mood fluctuations regarding activities and relationships:
  Red – angry, frustrated or embarrassed.
  White – tired and lacking energy.
  Yellow – fed up.
  Green – envious.
  Orange – annoyed at being angry, frustrated or embarrassed.
  Blue / black – agonised and offended.
- Other unnatural states are:
  – Sunken insteps: drained and exhausted.
  – Swollen insteps: weighed down and burdened. Overcome by the enormity of life's circumstances.
  – Wrinkled upper insteps: concerned about actions.
  – Wrinkled lower insteps: worried about associations.
  – Crossed lines: at crossroads.
  – Netted lines: feeling trapped.

- Deep vertical lines: Pulled in two directions or keeping personal ideas separate from social and family expectations in matters concerning activities and/or relationships.
- Irregular lines: havoc and confusion.

Many other significant markings can be present. All indicate a need to find direction and inner peace.

Digestive, adrenal and ——— kidney ailments eased ——— through reflexology

For any disorder, a complete reflexology massage is required, with the greatest emphasis being on:

- nervous system and solar plexus reflexes to calm the mind and relieve pain, anxiety and fear
- endocrine gland reflexes to soothe the emotions and create inner harmony
- affected glands or organ reflexes to relax the distressed area and ease the symptoms of dis-ease.

The following also include middle back disorders.

Abdominal cramps   Replaces the gripping fear and anxiety about activities or relationships and the consequences thereof with self-confidence.

Addictions   Inflates self-image and eliminates the need for self-destructive behavioural patterns.

Addison's disease   Provides fortification through appreciation of personal assets.

Adrenal disorders   Boosts inner strength by understanding self-worth.

Alcoholism   Encourages acceptance of the self, regardless of the opinions of others, and removes the need to drown sorrows.

Anorexia   Provides a purpose to exist and gives an incentive to nourish mind, body and soul for the benefit of all concerned.

Appendicitis   Replaces with understanding and empathy the fear and frustration of past communications.

Appetite   Provides a natural need for life sustenance.

Belching   Calms the speed of life.

Bowel disorders   Releases individuals from the perceived pressure of high achievement by eliminating wasted ideas and emotions threatening present relationships and personal security.

Bulimia   Provides the courage to accept all aspects of life and do all that is required without feeling overwhelmed, threatened or inadequate.

Cellulite   Dismisses perceived obstructions and blockages through believing in personal abilities.

Cholecystitis (inflammation of the gall bladder)   Replaces the bitterness and resentment of past actions with understanding and self-forgiveness.

Colic   If the sufferer is a baby, massage the mother's feet to pacify maternal irritability, intolerance and impatience.

Colitis   Soothes inflamed feelings at being inappropriately hassled through the release of old relationships once and for all.

Colon disorders   Allows self-acceptance to dispel the dread of failure through the expulsion of life's remnants.

Constipation   Encourages the release of burdensome belief systems that threaten personal security.

Diabetes   Occurs eighteen months to two years after the upset of a traumatic event, such as a death or break-up, which temporarily removes the joy of living. New opportunities in the changed situation reinstate hope and eventual happiness.

Diarrhoea   Eliminates the need to run away when feeling fearful or rejected.

Haemorrhoids   Removes discontent at being encumbered, pressurised, strained or suppressed.

Hypoglycaemia   Re-energises the whole with renewed enthusiasm for full enjoyment of life.

Liver disorders   Creates inner harmony by calming fiery emotions, profound dissatisfaction and suppressed guilt. Dismisses the need to be aggressive and continually critical of others.

Malabsorption syndrome   Replenishes the mind, body and soul through absorption of the beneficial aspects of relationships and improved communication.

Middle back problems   Releases perceived guilt at lack of support regarding activities and/or relationships and replaces it with the wisdom derived from the experiences of life.

Nephritis Eliminates anger and frustration at continual disappointments.

Overweight Removes the perceived need to cover up, reject, conceal or protect one's true self.

Pancreatitis Replaces resentment at the lack of sweetness and joy in personal activities with understanding.

Peptic ulcer Restores belief in personal aptitude so that fear of inadequacy no longer eats away at oneself.

Small intestine disorders Facilitates the absorption of the beneficial aspects of life by boosting self-esteem and self-worth.

Solar plexus Calms the 'abdominal brain' so that it is less sensitive and no longer overreacts to upsetting, distressing and nerve-racking situations.

Spastic colon Relieves the pressure and irritability of meeting self-imposed expectations by feeling secure.

Spleen disorders Reinstates balance, faith and appreciation in all activities.

Starvation Replaces thoughts and feelings of deprivation and martyrdom with renewed self-worth.

Stomach upsets Creates inner tranquillity by removing the upset and uncertainty of new circumstances and the fear of not coping.

Vomiting Encourages the acceptance of perceivably repulsive situations that are difficult to stomach through understanding the growth experience involved.

11
THE HEELS

The heels mirror the:

- pelvic bones
- lower back
- hands
- feet
- lower urinary system
- reproductive glands and organs.

They reflect:

- basic security
- mobility
- personal growth
- individual development.

Position of the reflexes on the heels and the effect of reflexology on these reflexes

The reflexes of the pelvic bone fill most of the heel surfaces and are also reflected onto the outer ankle-bones (Figure 89). Through reflexology they provide a solid foundation for self-development.

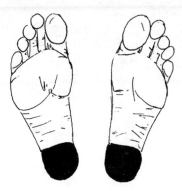

Figure 89   Pelvic bone reflexes

The hip joint reflexes are bony swellings immediately beneath the outer ankle-bone (Figure 90). Massage provides the impetus and force to move ahead with ease.

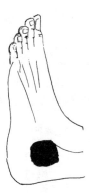

Figure 90   Hip joint reflexes

The hand reflexes are softer swellings on the tops of both feet in front of the outer ankle bones (Figure 91). Reflexology facilitates and encourages confidence in handling the experiences in life.

The feet are reflected onto the lower edges of the heel pads (Figure 92), as well as onto both outer surfaces, beneath the outer ankle-bones (Figure 93). Through reflexology, feet are able to provide stability and mobility for personal security, growth and development.

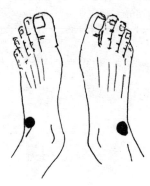

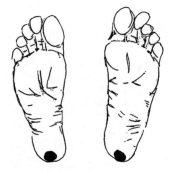

Figure 91   Hand reflexes

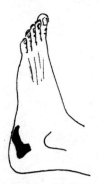

Figure 92   Reflexes of the feet on the heel pads

Figure 93   Reflexes of the feet on the sides of the heels

The reflexes of the reproductive organs and glands are reflected onto the inner surfaces of both ankles (Figures 94 and 95). The female

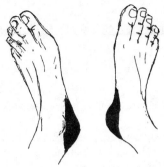

Figure 94 Male reproductive organs and glands reflexes

organs and glands also spread across the lower insteps on the soles of the feet (Figure 68). Massage of reproductive organs and glands reflexes encourages acceptance of distinctive personal gender and sexual characteristics.

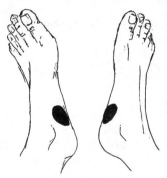

Figure 95 Female reproductive organs reflexes

The bony ridges that curve under the inner ankle-bones are the lower back reflexes (see Figure 100) and reflect the perceived security and backing required to expand and explore new horizons, which can be strengthened by massaging these reflexes.

The buttock reflexes, on the rounded mounds beneath the outer ankle-bones, reflect the amount of power and control over personal direction. Flabby buttocks feel out of control and reliant on others for security, whilst exceptionally taut buttocks keep a tight rein on affairs.

❝ Circumstances do not determine **what** we are, they only reveal **who** we are! ❞

—— Impact of tension on the heels ——

Heels are often heavy from not being able to get ahead due to:

- the constraints of limited family and social laws that deny individuals the opportunity to fully realise and develop personal talents.
- conditioned belief systems that create a subconscious or conscious fear of venturing into the unknown and of change.
- the perceived lack of finances preventing individuals from participating in educational or experimental pursuits for personal growth.

Doubt, uncertainty and lack of courage stunt progress and growth, physically, emotionally and spiritually, leading to extreme frustration and insecurity. This is reflected on the feet accordingly:

- pelvic bone reflexes, on the heels, contract, becoming less effective as shock absorbers
- hip reflexes, beneath the outer ankle-bones, swell, inhibiting the free flow of movement
- hand reflexes:
  - bulge with the enormity of handling demanding situations.
  - subside when fearful or dubious about dealings.
- feet reflexes, on the heel pads and outer ankle surfaces, bulge when life is perceived to be a drag or heavy going.
- male reproductive organs and glands reflexes:
  - develop broken blood vessels or bruises when masculinity or the male role is threatened
  - protrude in search of recognition of masculine qualities
  - deflate when the male ego has been knocked.
- vaginal reflexes:
  - expand when overwhelmed by perceived demands made because of femineity
  - are covered with broken blood vessels or bruised due to perceived sexual harassment and abuse, either physical or emotional.

- lower back reflexes:
  - distend with concern for financial matters
  - collapse when there are insufficient funds to provide support or when there is a drain on personal resources.

Reflexology massage of the heel reflexes

Step 1

- Place the thumbs or third fingers on the outer, upper edge of both heel pads and gently massage with the caterpillar or rotation technique in horizontal strips beneath the insteps.

Step 2

- Repeat Step 1 fractionally lower down the heels and continue to do so until both heel pads have been thoroughly massaged (Figure 96).

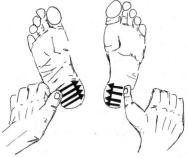

Figure 96   Massaging the heel pads

Step 3

- Place the thumbs or third fingers on the outer, upper edges of both heels but this time slide the digits in vertical strips down the outside edges of the heels in a milking movement (Figure 97).

- Repeat the milking movement placing the digits fractionally further onto the heel pads. Slide the digits in vertical strips from top to bottom in a milking movement.

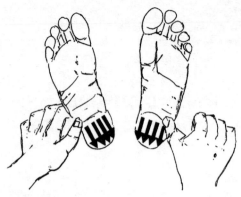

Figure 97 Milking the heel pads

- Continue to milk these reflexes moving the digits further and further along the heel pads to the inner heel edges until completely milked.
- Feather stroke the heel pads from top to bottom, starting on the outer and finishing on the inner edges.

Step 4

- Visualise imaginary lines from the bases of both heels to the tips of the third toes.
- With minimal contact, rest the tips of both third fingers or both thumbs at the bottoms of the imaginary lines on the bases of both heels (Figure 98). Stay a while.

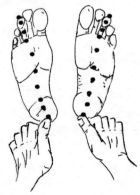

Figure 98 Balancing the energies

- Now move up the imaginary lines to lightly touch the centres of the heel pads and hold for a few seconds.
- Continue to move up the imaginary lines, making light contact: at the junctions of the insteps and heels; in the centres of the insteps; at the solar plexus reflexes; in the centres of the balls; on the necks of the third toes; in the centre of the pads of the third toes; on the tips of the third toes.
- This technique balances the energies and is exceptionally uplifting and rejuvenating. Since it is so powerful, it needs to be applied with tremendous love and sensitivity.

Step 5

- Now massage the outer triangular areas of the heels, beneath the outside ankle-bones, first with the caterpillar or rotation movement then with the milking technique and finally feather stroking, all towards the recipient (Figure 99).
- The outer heels contain the buttock and feet reflexes.

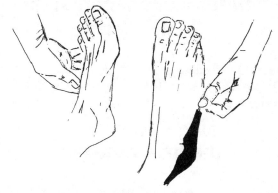

Figure 99 Massaging buttock and foot reflexes

Step 6

- Place both thumbs on the bony ridges on the insides of both feet where the insteps meet the heels (Figure 100).
- Massage the bony ridges along the bases of both inner ankles, first with the caterpillar or rotation techniques, then with the milking action and finally with the feather stroke movement.
- These are the lower spine and vertebral reflexes.

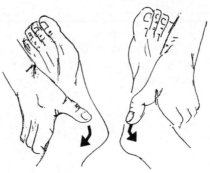

Figure 100 Massaging the lower spine reflexes

Stroke both feet, top and bottom, from toes to ankles, and then finish the reflexology massage with the finale.

❝ A change of life is only two feet away. ❞

Natural characteristics of the heels

The heels are naturally flesh-coloured rotund mounds, like firm, pliable cushions, that provide a spring to the step and act as shock absorbers.

Altered states of the heel reflexes

Self-imposed limitations are immediately reflected onto the heels:

Cracked heel pads – pulled in many directions.
Hardened heel pads – difficulty in moving ahead.
Hardened rims – digging the heels in.
Heavy heel pads – making progress is heavy going.
Painful heel pads – unhappy about personal growth and development.
Rough heel pads – perceives a rough path.
Spongy heel pads – gives in too easily.
Bruised heel pads – wounded at direction in life or the lack of it.

The colour of the skin indicates the emotion concerned (see page 118).

❝ At any point in time there are many future possibilities – we can choose any one and still change direction en route. ❞

Reproductive, skeletal, —— muscular and urinary ailments —— eased through reflexology

For any disorder, a complete reflexology massage is required, with greater emphasis on:

- nervous system and solar plexus reflexes to calm the mind and relieve pain, anxiety and fear
- endocrine gland reflexes to soothe the emotions and create inner harmony
- affected gland or organ reflexes to relax the distressed area and ease the symptoms of dis-ease.

Amenorrhoea Removes the need to withdraw from femineity by realising the beauty of female energy.

Anal disorders Eliminates wasted emotions to promote and encourage progress.

Ankle disorders Increases flexibility and the ability to adapt to the pleasure of life's ups and downs.

Anorectal bleeding Releases the sadness of having little or no basic backing or support.

Arms Strengthens the ability and capacity to embrace the fullness of life.

Bed wetting Replaces insecure foundations and lack of control with inner security.

Birth defects The type of defect reveals extreme anxiety of the mother during pregnancy. Reflexology during pregnancy decreases this eventuality. Perceived inherited disorders are adopted belief systems that no longer have value.

Bone Bolsters inner strength and personal support:
- Broken or fractured bone: resistance to unreasonable control and the break away from limiting circumstances is eased.
- Bone deformity: the bone is liberated from perceived pressures and strictness.

Bursitis   Soothes inflamed thoughts and provides flexibility to move ahead in the required direction.

Buttocks   Assists in regaining power, security and basic supports for life.

Cystitis   Expels frustration and anger of feeling continually discontented in holding onto wasted emotions that threaten personal security.

Lower back pain   Enriches mind, body and soul by dissipating the hurt at not feeling secure, particularly financially.

❛ Those who expect the best in life will be fulfilled, with testing points along the way to enrich life's experiences. ❜

12

THE FINALE

Body, mind and soul should be completely relaxed and at ease by now, making it an ideal time to stretch and manipulate both feet for greater flexibility and expansion of the whole.

Step 1

- Gently pull both little toes simultaneously (Figure 101), then the fourth toes, followed by the third and second toes, and finally the two big toes.
- Hold the pull for longer on the big toes, especially for neck tension, headaches or back disorders.

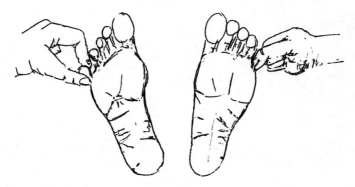

Figure 101   Pulling the toes

Step 2

- Lightly support the base of the right little toe with the left thumb and index finger.
- Hold the right little toe between the right thumb and index finger (Figure 102).
- Rotate the little toe, first anticlockwise, then clockwise.
- Then pivot the fourth right toe, followed by the rest of the toes on the right foot.

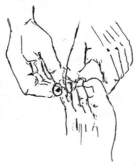

Figure 102   Rotating the toes

- Repeat on the left foot, rotating first the left little toe and finishing with the left big toe.
- Extra attention, particularly to the big toes, effectively reduces neck stiffness and tension.

Step 3

- Embrace the upper part of the right foot with the palms of the hands placed either side (Figure 103).
- Gently roll the foot by moving the hands alternately up and down.
- Repeat on the left foot.

Step 4

- With both hands placed on top of both feet, gently but firmly stretch the feet downwards (Figure 104).

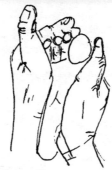

Figure 103   Rolling the upper part of the foot

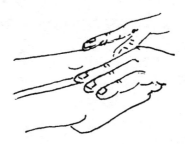

Figure 104   Stretching the feet down

Step 5

- Now place the palms of the hands flat against the soles of both feet and gradually ease them upwards (Figure 105).

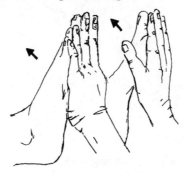

Figure 105   Pushing the feet upwards

Step 6

- Support the right heel with the left hand and use the right hand to circulate the right foot, first anticlockwise and then clockwise (Figure 106).
- Change hands and repeat on the left foot.

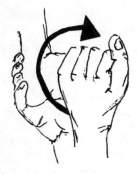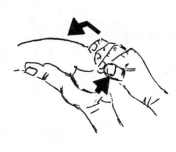

Figure 106   Circling the feet

Step 7

- Place both thumbs beneath the right little toe neck with the fingers immediately opposite, on top of the feet (Figure 107).
- Gently push the thumbs up whilst lightly stretching the tops of the feet downwards with the fingers.

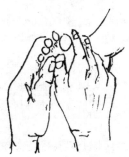

Figure 107   Manipulating the feet

- Continue this movement all the way down the soles, from top to bottom, beneath the right little toe.

- Repeat down the length of the sole beneath the fourth toe and all the other toes until the right foot has been completely manipulated.
- Loosen the left foot in the same way.

Step 8

- The reflexology sequence is completed with the massage of the solar plexus reflexes (page 92) for at least one minute.
- Finally gently stroke first the right and then the left foot thoroughly before covering the feet with the sheet or blanket.
- Hold the covered feet and in a soft voice invite the recipient to take in three deep breaths to ease themselves out of the alpha state of consciousness.
- Encourage them to stay lying flat and surface in their own time.
- Provide a glass of purified water and recommend that plenty of water is consumed for at least 24 hours to flush out the systems.
- Reassure them that any reaction (page 40) is an excellent sign of detoxification, purification and healing.
- Advise the recipient to wrap up warmly after a reflexology massage, especially if it is cold, since tremendous heat can be lost when so relaxed.

———— General ailments ————

Several ailments affect all bodily systems or differing parts at various stages. To assess the position of affected reflexes refer to the foot chart on page 22.

Babies or children mirror uneasiness within the parent, particularly the mother, so ideally all family members should receive reflexology. As the adults improve, so the offspring will reflect the recovery.

——— General ailments eased ——— through reflexology

For any disorder, a complete reflexology massage is required, with emphasis on:

- nervous system and solar plexus reflexes to calm the mind and relieve pain, anxiety and fear
- endocrine gland reflexes to soothe the emotions and create inner harmony
- affected gland or organ reflexes to relax the distressed area and ease the symptoms of dis-ease.

Abscess Accumulated hurts and inflamed emotions surface for eventual release and relief from past traumas.

Accidents Dissipates the reckless need to go headlong into situations.

Arthritis Replace rigidity and uncertainty with security and flexibility, with the realisation that the perfect life starts when we stop wanting a better one.

Bites Provides protection against perceived outside attack which draws on personal substance.

Blisters Soothes friction that comes to a head.

Body odour Calms nervousness and boosts self-confidence.

Boils Brings to a head frustrating aspects that have got under the skin.

Bruises Eases emotional knocks in life, using them as knocks of opportunity for self-development.

Burns Releases extreme anger and frustration that has surfaced.

Callouses Removes the need to cover up, protect or conceal true thoughts and emotions, by boosting belief in personal abilities.

Cancer Encourages open expression of contained feelings to calm inner havoc and distorted emotions.

Candida Centres the individual so that there is no longer frustration at being pulled in many directions to please others, but instead nurtures the self for the benefit of all.

Carbuncle Brings to a head and releases repressed anger and frustration of life circumstances that get under the skin.

Childhood diseases Dismisses the childlike behaviour of the parent.

Chills Encourages the individual to come in from the cold and stop withdrawing into oneself.

Colds Urges mind, body and soul to exonerate outdated belief systems and sad, irritating thoughts to make way for new, exciting concepts.

Congestion Relaxes the musculature to loosen and let go of congested emotions for free flow and distribution of energy and enthusiasm throughout the whole.

Corns Removes the perceived need to protect personal concepts from being trampled on or from blocking out hurtful aspects.

Cramp Eases gripping fear.

Cuts Creates inner peace so that there is no longer a feeling of being cut up and torn apart.

Cysts Eliminates the need to gain attention and recognition of accumulated hurts and injured feelings.

Eczema Calms emotional turmoil of irritants that erupt under the skin.

Fatigue Fills the whole with an enthusiasm for life that defies boredom and tiredness.

Fever Encourages heated emotions to surface and dissipate.

Fever blisters Increases tolerance to fiery emotions that cause friction.

Fibroid cysts Relaxes the tight grip on accumulated hurts, allowing them to escape and disappear.

Fistula Dissipates the need to form emotional escape routes.

Fungi Refuses to allow old emotions to dwell and hurt the body.

Gangrene Restores a vibrant blood flow to the deprived area by eliminating morbid thoughts.

Glandular diseases Enhances the distribution of lively thoughts and ideas for the well-being of the whole.

Gout Dismisses the burning need to dominate, and replaces anger and impatience with lenience.

Infection, inflammation Soothes inflamed, infuriating emotions.

Influenza Disposes of mass negativity and beliefs that cause widespread pain and irritability.

Itching Meets the innate desire to move ahead or escape from irritating circumstances.

Multiple sclerosis Dissolves the strictness of having to conform to rigid belief systems.

Muscular disorders Facilitates moving ahead with ease.

Nail biting Restores confidence in handling life.

Numbness Fills the whole with renewed sensitivity and unconditional love for oneself and others.

Oedema Expels old emotions that weigh heavily on the mind, body and soul.

Pain Banishes the hurt of inadequacy or criticism.

Parasites Sets free those who are perceived to be drawing on personal resources.

Plantar wart Dissipates frustration and anger at the direction of life.

Rheumatism   Dissolves past resentment and bitterness.

Sclerosis   Liberates the whole from an intense desire to control.

Shingles   Relinquishes the hurt and pain at the inadequacy of putting personal ideas into action.

Skin disorders   Pacifies the whole so that life does not get under the skin.

Snoring   Frees deep-seated emotions that have been kept close to the chest.

Spinal curvature   Reinforces overall support and backing.

Swelling   Liberates entrapped emotions.

Twitching   Boosts self-esteem and self-confidence by removing anxiety and fear of the consequences.

Ulcers   Reinstates belief in oneself.

Warts   Removes the need to project concepts of self-hate and ugliness.

Weakness   Provides inner strength to enjoy the fullness of life.

Wounds   Heals emotional hurts.

❛ Live well for today,
For yesterday is but a dream,
And tomorrow but a vision.

But today well lived
Makes every yesterday a dream of happiness,
And every tomorrow a vision of hope. ❜

CONCLUSION

Reflexology today and in the future

Reflexology, once valued as a healing medium, became less popular during the scientific revolution around 250 years ago. Like many other concepts that linked the mind, body and soul, it was dismissed as unscientific. The body then became treated as some kind of sophisticated machine that could only be serviced and maintained by highly trained, specialised personnel.

With armour-plated defence mechanisms and mass belief conditioning it was inevitable that dis-ease and unrest would become widespread. The resultant panic and hysteria worldwide arises from having lost touch with our true selves, as well as with the abundance of the universe.

Boredom, emptiness and world-weariness are symptoms of materialism which impoverishes the mind and soul. Masses are starved and deprived of a deeper meaning to life that cannot be discovered through systematic, scientific research.

Increasing desperation from the realisation that complete solutions are not available in the physical world alone has generated renewed interest in ancient healing practices, such as reflexology. Many turn to these ancient forms of therapy when all else has failed and are amazed at the effectiveness.

The trend to look for other points of view is expanding with discovery that inner peace and harmony are possible, even in these distressing times of violence, confusion and fear. More people are taking responsibility for their health and well-being, and in so doing are improving the world through healing themselves by natural means.

Reflexology liberates individuals from self-imposed restrictions and encourages people to step ahead to a more fulfilling and meaningful way of life.

❛ There is inside us, all of the potential to be whatever we wish to be,
All of the energy to do whatever we would like to do.
If we imagine ourselves as we would like to be,
Doing what we want to do,
And each day take a step towards our dream,
Although at times it may seem impossible to continue holding
onto that dream,
One day we shall awake
To find that we are the person we dreamed of,
Doing what we wanted to do,
Simply because we had the courage
To believe in our potential And hold onto our dream. ❜

AUTHOR'S FOOTNOTE

The verses and sayings used in this book are not original or attributable; they have been quoted and used by many peoples for centuries.

> ❛ No thought is an original thought,
> And no utterance an original utterance. ❜

The unconditional sharing of universal knowledge allows us to become greater, more enlightened souls.

May all your dreams come true!

FURTHER READING

The author, Chris Stormer, is a world acclaimed authority on reflexology. Her previous books are enjoyed by those with a general interest in this fascinating form of healing and are also used as text and hand books in Reflexology and Healing Establishments and Training Centres throughout the world. To supplement the information in this book obtain copies of:

Reflexology – Headway Lifeguides 0 340 55594 7

Reflexology – The Definitive Guide 0 340 62038 2

Language of the Feet 0 340 64345 5

All books, published by Hodder & Stoughton, London, are available through most literary outlets. If sold out and therefore not immediately available, ask the bookstore to place an order for you.

APPENDIX 1

__ Healing enhanced through the __ use of aromatherapy oils

The sensuous aspect of aromatherapy oils has a therapeutic effect on mind, body and soul. A mixture of one to three oils with approximately 30 ml of almond oil can be rubbed into the feet during or at the end of the massage to enhance the effect of reflexology.

Uplifting oils To boost confidence, ease depression and eliminate moodiness. Examples are clary sage, jasmine and grapefruit.

Regulating oils To relieve anxiety and re-establish equilibrium. Examples are bergamot, frankincense, geranium and rosewood.

Stimulating oils To strengthen concentration, clear the mind and improve memory. Examples are lemon, peppermint, rosemary and black pepper.

Invigorationg oils To fill the whole with enthusiasm and interest and strengthen the immune system. Examples are cardamom, juniper, rosemary and lemongrass.

Soothing oils To increase levels of tolerance, improve sleep patterns and calm the mind. Examples are camomile, lavender, marjoram and orange blossom.

Aphrodisiac oils To strengthen relationships and boost self-esteem. Examples are jasmine, clary sage, patchouli and ylang ylang.

There are many other valuable aromatherapy oils that can be used to accelerate healing. Specialised books are filled with a wealth of information on the subject.

APPENDIX 2

The vibration of colours for inner harmony

Visualisation of colours during reflexology massage alters the vibrational tone of healing energies absorbed by the body. The resultant fine tuning reconnects mind, body and soul for overall harmony and peace.

The following guide recommends colours that can be visualised during reflexology massage of the various areas on the feet. Should another colour come to mind, or if the colour changes, stay with the adjustment since this is the vibration required.

Red on the heels provides security, mobility and enthusiasm for individual growth and development. 'See red' when obstacles are perceived to obstruct personal actualisation.

Orange on the lower insteps communicates the joy at feeling secure within relationships, so making life pleasurable.

Yellow on the upper insteps re-establishes control knowing that, with stability and affinity, actions benefit all those concerned.

Green on the balls of the feet harmonises internal and external relationships with personal achievements, interactions and security, enhancing unconditional love for oneself and others.

Blue on the toe necks calms and clarifies the mind and body for the open and honest expression of the soul.

Purple on the toes raises the level of consciousness for clarity of thought, peace of mind, emotional harmony and body alignment.

APPENDIX 3

Music to relax body, mind and soul

The abundance of beautiful music available today makes it impossible to mention it all, especially when taking into consideration, personal preferences. Here are a few suggestions:

- Dolphin and whale music, especially beneficial for pregnancy and childbirth and for restless or disturbed souls.
- Natural sounds such as the wind, sea, waterfalls, birdsong and so on. Examples:
  - *Wilderness* by Tony O'Connor
  - *Wetland Symphony* by Ducks Unlimited Canada.
- Ethnic music using traditional instruments. Examples:
  - *Cusco, Apurimac II. Return to ancient America*
  - *Eagle* by Medwyn Goodall
  - *Uluru* by Tony O'Connor.
- Pan flutes. Example:
  - *In Touch* by Tony O'Connor.
- Electrical harp. Examples:
  - *Dream Spiral* by Hilary Stagg.
- Other suggestions:
  - *Gifts of the Angels* by Steven Halpern
  - *Bushland Dreaming* by Tony O'Connor
  - *Rhythmist; Inner Tides; Lunar Reflections* by Ian Cameron Smith.

REFLEXOLOGY CENTRES AND TRAINING ORGANISERS

Worldwide

The International Council of
    Reflexology Therapists
Barbara Mosier
PO Box 621963
Littleton CO 80162
USA
Facsimile: (303) 904 0460

America

Elaine Gordon
PO Box 732
Westside Station
Worcester
Mass 01602
Telephone/Facsimile: (508) 793 1571

Australia

Brisbane

Catherine Pretorius
RASA (Australia)
73 Illawong Way
Karand Downs 4306
Telephone/Facsimile: (07) 201 0680

Melbourne

Dee Leamon
Australian School of Reflexology
    and Relaxation
165 Progress Road
Eltham North
Victoria 3095
Telephone: (03) 439 6217/572 2214
Facsimile: (03) 571 0629

Perth

Joan Cass
RASA Organiser
75 Fifth Ave
Rossmoyne
Western Australia
Telephone: (09) 457 3117
Facsimile: (09) 332 3940

Sydney

Sue Ehinger
The Australian School of Reflexology
15 Kedumba Crescent
Turramurra 2074
New South Wales
Telephone: (02) 988 3881
Facsimile: (02) 44 5363

Sue Enzer
Soul to Sole Reflexology
1599A Pacific Highway
Wahroonga 2076
New South Wales
Telephone: (02) 489 4941/015 274 958

Tasmania

Pam Kelly
Tasmanian School of Reflexology and
    Natural Therapies
80 Junction Street
Launceston 7249
Telephone: (003) 44 6620
Facsimile: (003) 44 9257

Canada

Jean-Louis Dube
11 Glen Cameron Road
Unit 4
Thornhill Crescent
Ontario L3T 4N3
Telephone: (905) 889 5900/(613)
    724 6021
Facsimile: (905) 889 7099/(613)
    724 6213

Ollie Bailey
32052 Sherwood Crescent
Clearbrook
British Columbia
Canada V2T 1C2
Telephone/Facsimile: (604) 859 3338

China

Hang Xiongwen
Chairman Professor
China Reflexology Association
PO Box 2002
Beijing 100026
P R China
Telephone: 506 8310
Facsimile: 506 8309

Egypt

Rawya El Gammal
19 Gabalaya Street
Zamalek
Cairo 11211.
Telephone: (202) 340 6167
Facsimile: (202) 341 1752

Greece

Rene Stravelaki
85 Alkionis 17562
P Fadiro
Athens
Telephone: (01) 984 1030
Facsimile: (01) 988 0310

Hong Kong

Nicole Wilson
19D Woodland Court
Lantau Island
Telephone: 2987 6557
Facsimile: 2521 6132

New Zealand

Alys Noyes
PO Box 5233
Regent Whangarai
Telephone: (025) 989770 (Work)
(09) 437000 (Home)

Emma Frommings
7 South Beach Road
Plummerton
Wellington
Telephone: (04) 233 8366 (Home)
(04) 233 9695 (Work)

Adrienne Bates
PO Box 519
Keri Keri.
Telephone: (09) 445 6132

South Africa

Chris Stormer
The Reflexology Academy of
Southern Africa
PO Box 1280
Rivonia 2128
Telephone: (011) 803 1552/803 5946
Facsimile: (011) 803 5946/803 9052

Gini Swiss
The Reflexology Academy of
Southern Africa (Natal)
PO Box 53
Bothas Hill 3660
Natal
Telephone: (031) 752 738
Facsimile: (031) 720 078

Gayl Hansen
The Cape College of Natural Healing
50 Windermere Road
Muizenberg
Cape Province
Telephone: (021) 788 8347

United Kingdom

England

Salvina Macari
The Little Grange School of
Reflexology
189 Canterbury Road
Westbrook
Margate
Kent CT9 5DA
Telephone: (01843) 295910

Ireland

Kathy Rea
Irish Council of Reflexology
Therapists
Lisburn
Co Antrim
Northern Ireland
Telephone/Facsimile: (01846) 677 806

Anthony Larkin
The Bayly School of Reflexology
(Ireland)
41 Parkfield
New Ross
County Wexford
Ireland
Telephone: (051) 22209

Scotland

Patrick McMenemy
17 Cairnwell Avenue
Mastrict
Aberdeen AB2 5SH
Telephone: (01224 697309

Trudi Schaller
Strathearn Holistic Centre
Western Road
Gleneagles
Perthshire PH2 1JL
Telephone: (01764) 684 365

Zimbabwe

Eileen Westley
Association of Complementary Health
   Practitioners of Zimbabwe
Box GD 362
Greendale
Harare

INDEX